Public Health

Power, Empowerment and Professional Practice
2nd Edition

Glenn Laverack

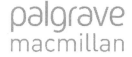

First edition published 2005
Reprinted once
Second edition published 2009 by
PALGRAVE MACMILLAN

Palgrave Macmillan in the UK is an imprint of Macmillan Publishers Limited, registered in England, company number 785998, of Houndmills, Basingstoke, Hampshire RG21 6XS.

Palgrave Macmillan in the US is a division of St Martin's Press LLC, 175 Fifth Avenue, New York, NY 10010.

Palgrave Macmillan is the global academic imprint of the above companies and has companies and representatives throughout the world.

Palgrave® and Macmillan® are registered trademarks in the United States, the United Kingdom, Europe and other countries.

ISBN 978-0-230-21798-0 paperback

This book is printed on paper suitable for recycling and made from fully managed and sustained forest sources. Logging, pulping and manufacturing processes are expected to conform to the environmental regulations of the country of origin.

A catalogue record for this book is available from the British Library.

A catalog record for this book is available from the Library of Congress.

Printed in Great Britain by the MPG Books Group, Bodmin and King's Lynn

Contents

List of tables, figures and boxes

■ Tables

■ Figures

■ Boxes

Acknowledgements

I would like to acknowledge the many people with whom I have had the privilege of working and exchanging ideas during the course of writing a second edition. In particular I would like to thank Dr Samson Tse, Kathleen Eskine-Shaw, Mary Strang and Linda Johnston for their insightful comments.

To Bernie Trude, who was a true friend and a very courageous person.

To my family, Elizabeth, Ben, Holly and Rebecca for their unconditional love and support.

Preface

This book is the second edition and builds on the first publication with new international case study material, new practical approaches and strategies for empowerment. The book has been written to meet the continued demand from Practitioners who want to work in a more empowering way and has an emphasis on the work of nurse Practitioners.

Public health always entails some power differential that can be best described in regard to the relationship between 'Practitioners' and their 'clients'. Practitioners are employed to deliver information, resources and services in public health programmes that are professionally led and have a predetermined agenda that does not always meet client needs. The clients are viewed as the recipients of the information, resources and services and as part of a programme in which they are expected to participate and towards which they are expected to contribute. In a top-down style of public health it is the Practitioner that has power-over the programme and their clients. Little wonder then that public health programmes have traditionally failed to close the gap in health status between different social and economic groups in society and may in fact have contributed, at least temporarily, to their share of inequality.

Empowerment, the means to attaining power, is a process of capacity building with the goal of bringing about social and political change in favour of the individuals, groups and communities seeking more control. The relationship between public health, civil society and social movements is an important one in this process and is discussed in this book. But to only view empowerment as a means of mass emancipation is to miss the point of public health and the majority of empowering opportunities that occur on a day-to-day basis. It is through these opportunities that Practitioners become involved with the poor, the marginalised or simply with concerned individuals, groups and community-based organisations that seek to gain more control over the problems that influence their lives and health.

It is those Practitioners who have the professional competencies to help their clients to gain control over their lives that will be best placed to work in an empowering way. I draw heavily on my own professional experience to share with the reader ways that I have found to be meaningful to help empower others. The book offers a gradual way forward rather than a radical reorientation of existing public health practice, a way that is more empowering for both the Practitioner and their clients. The challenge to the reader is to use the creative ways in this book to enable the public health agencies with whom they work to better empower individuals, groups and communities.

GLENN LAVERACK, Auckland, New Zealand.

An overview of the book

This book has four main purposes:

1. To provide the reader with a theoretical understanding of the concepts of power and empowerment in Chapters 1 and 2.
2. To introduce the reader to practical approaches for helping individuals, groups and communities to gain power in Chapters 3, 4, 5 and 6.
3. To provide the reader with a practical means to build, measure and visually represent community empowerment in Chapter 7.
4. To bring together the main themes of the book and to discuss what the future of public health programming will have to look like to be more successful in achieving its goals in Chapter 8.

■ Chapter 1   Power, empowerment and public health practice in context

Chapter 1 provides an introduction to the evolution of the concept of empowerment within public health practice. The different roles of the public health Practitioner and the sometimes problematic relationship that they have with their clients and with other professionals are discussed. Chapter 1 introduces the reader to the influence of bureaucratic settings, in which most public health Practitioners work, the hegemony of the medical profession, lay epidemiology and the fragmentation of professional practice. Chapter 1 also provides an introduction to how our professional interpretation of public health is a function of our understanding of the concept of health.

■ Chapter 2   Power and empowerment

Chapter 2 moves the reader into the territory of how power, powerlessness and empowerment are central to public health practice. The purpose is to make these complex concepts, and the way in which they interact, more understandable in a practical sense to Practitioners. Chapter 2 also discusses the social and cultural perceptions of power and empowerment and the implications that this can have for public health practice.

■ Chapter 3   Empowerment and public health programming

Chapter 3 includes a discussion of the tensions that exist in public health programming between 'top-down' and 'bottom-up' approaches and a way to resolve this issue through 'parallel-tracking' using the example of maternal and newborn health. Chapter 3 also discusses the importance of problem assessment and resolving conflict when working with communities and offers practical solutions to each of these areas in a programme context.

■ Chapter 4   Helping individuals to gain power

Chapter 4 addresses how public health Practitioners can better work with individuals to help them to gain power, and in particular, by becoming more effective communicators, by increasing the critical awareness of their clients and by fostering an empowering working relationship. Chapter 4 also discusses the power of professional language and how this can influence the professional-client relationship.

■ Chapter 5   Helping groups and communities to gain power

Chapter 5 addresses those aspects of empowerment that enhance the ability of groups and communities to better organise and mobilise themselves towards gaining power. Chapter 5 clarifies the concepts of community and community empowerment and offers a framework for helping groups and communities to gain more power, including the important role of social movements, towards social and political action.

■ Chapter 6   Helping marginalised people to gain power

Chapter 6 takes the discussion of community empowerment further to examine how Practitioners can help marginalised people to gain power. In particular, Chapter 6 provides two case study examples. The first is of how indigenous communities in Australia were helped to gain control of local health service delivery. The second is how Practitioners can work with Chinese migrants to improve health outcomes by preventing injuries and by promoting health care and rehabilitation services.

■ Chapter 7   The measurement and visual representation of community empowerment

Chapter 7 discusses the importance of and provides the means to collecting and analysing qualitative information as an important professional competence for the measurement of community empowerment. The measurement of community empowerment and its visual representation is then discussed using a case study example of gaining control over local resources in Thailand.

■ Chapter 8   The future of public health programming

Finally, Chapter 8 discusses what the future of public health programming will have to look like in order to be more empowering and more successful in achieving its goals. To do this public health programming will have to find better ways of engaging with communities to share their priorities, systematically build community capacity, develop more flexible funding mechanisms, evaluate and be creative to expand on successful local initiatives.

Chapter 1

Power, empowerment and public health practice in context

■ Introduction

Public health is an approach that aims to promote health, prevent disease, treat illnesses, prolong valued life, care for the infirm and to provide health services. Traditionally, such goals of public health have been used to curb the spread of infectious diseases and to protect the well-being of the general population whilst others see a much greater role in regulation and reducing inequalities in health (Baggott, 2000). The range of goals also means that the term 'public health' is used to cover a number of specialist areas including environmental health, nursing and health promotion. Not surprisingly, public health remains a contested and contradictory term given the wide range of competing perspectives, priorities and services that it claims to deliver.

The different interests within public health help to shape what it looks like and the directions it takes as a professional practice by competing for limited resources, the control over decisions and the development of national policies. Public health also involves 'communities' and incorporates methods that connect collective action to the broader aims of political influence. Power and empowerment are key concepts to a public health practice that seeks to redress inequalities in health and to change the determinants of health through collective and community-based action.

In practice, public health still belongs primarily to people employed in the health sector, in the sense that it provides these workers with some conceptual models, professional legitimacy and resources. These people may be titled 'public health promoters' or 'health practitioners' while many more who look to the idea of public health occupy jobs such as health visitors, nurses and doctors. In this book, I refer to all these people as the 'Practitioner(s)'.

As a profession, public health is largely controlled by government departments, private sector agencies or Non-Governmental Organisations (NGOs) who employ Practitioners as 'professionals' to engage in programmes designed to improve or maintain the health of individuals, groups and communities. Professional groups within public health are expected to display a specialisation of knowledge, technical competence, social responsibility and services. Their level of professionalism is attained through education, specialised training, the testing of competence by formal examinations, the membership of a professional organisation and the inclusion of a professional code of practice (Turner and Samson, 1995).

Public health always entails some power relationship between different stake-holders, primarily between Practitioners and their clients. Practitioners are employed to deliver information, resources and services and are often seen as an outside agent to the people who are their clients. The term 'clients' covers the range of people who act as the recipients of the information, resources and services being delivered to promote health, for example, pregnant women, school children, the unemployed and concerned groups of individuals such as residents or organisations who have been formed to address a specific issue. I intentionally use the terms 'Practitioners' and 'clients' because they help to demonstrate the unbalanced power relationship that exists in public health practice.

One role of the Practitioner has traditionally been as an enforcer of public health legislation, for example, the Environmental Health Officer or 'Sanitary Policeman'. The role has been supported by much of the work of environmental health departments that are concerned with inspection, licensing, complaint investigations and legal proceedings. An enforcement of the wide range of public health, health protection and food safety legislation by Practitioners has been seen to be necessary to maintain a healthy and safe environment in the home, at work and during recreation. The role of the public health enforcer has helped to establish the image of some Practitioners as that of professionals with power-over their clients through the use of legislative controls.

Another role of the Practitioner has been concerned with education, training and specialist services, for example, as that of a nurse providing advice to a group of young mothers or providing treatment to their patients. This role has helped to broaden the image of the Practitioner as a health professional with 'expert' power and access to superior technical resources, skills and knowledge.

There is a further role of Practitioners, one that has developed more recently and that is complementary to their roles as enforcers, educators and specialists. It is an important role that has been largely overlooked because many Practitioners do not understand how their day-to-day work can be empowering for their clients. At the heart of this role is the ability of the Practitioners to transform their own power (access to information, resources and expertise) to a power-with relationship in which their clients are helped to gain more power. The outcome is that individuals, groups and communities are helped to gain greater control over decision making and access to available resources in regard to public health issues. I discuss this in detail in Chapter 2.

One of the main tensions that Practitioners face in an empowering approach to public health practice is whether their clients actually want to be empowered. Public health practice is traditionally professionally led, for example, it is the Practitioner or the agency that employs them that selects the clients and the methods to be used in a programme. The initiation of the empowerment process and the enthusiasm for its direction is also often led by the Practitioner. This is contradictory to an empowering approach in which the issue to be addressed and the means of reaching an empowered solution are the responsibility of the clients and not the Practitioner.

Some clients may not want to be empowered. People, especially if they have lived in powerless circumstances, may feel that they do not have the right or do not possess the motivation to empower themselves. Likewise, some Practitioners may feel powerlessness in their own work setting and in Chapter 4 I discuss ways in which Practitioners can overcome powerlessness in a professional context. In addition, some individuals and groups such as the mentally ill or people with an addiction may not have the ability to organise and mobilise themselves towards empowerment. What must be remembered is that power cannot be given to people but must be gained or seized by those who want it. The right or choice to be empowered essentially rests with the individual or group and the role of the Practitioner is to encourage their clients to take greater responsibility and control over their lives. For those people who cannot or who refuse to take responsibility then public health practice may have to intervene and resort to other means, for example, policy and legislation, to protect the general population from the spread of an infectious disease.

In this book I argue that Practitioners can and often do play an important role in facilitating change in their clients, either on a one-to-one basis or through working with groups and communities, to take greater control of their lives. Practitioners, who are in a position of relative power, work to help their clients, who are in a relatively powerless position, for example, by providing resources and skills, education and advisory services and by using their professional influence to legitimise community concerns. To achieve this Practitioners must work with other professionals and agencies, both public and private, such as education, housing and social services, if they are to develop effective strategies. Public health is also a product of a global market and strategies must increasingly cross international as well as organisational boundaries.

Practitioners must be flexible in their approach to working with clients whose abilities and competencies may have to be developed. The Practitioner may be initially tempted not to involve their clients and may undertake the responsibility of planning and implementation. The reason for this is usually to ensure that programmes are in place in time to meet deadlines. Participation can be compromised and in the longer-term the programme has far less chance of success. The importance of participation can be illustrated by a programme with women's groups in a poor rural population in Nepal which led to a reduction in neonatal and maternal mortality. The women in the intervention clusters were found to have antenatal care, institutional delivery, trained birth attendance and more hygienic care and that this led to an improvement in birth outcomes. By participating in groups the women were better able to define, analyse and then, through the support of others, articulate and act on their concerns around childbirth. The advantage of participation was that it strengthened social networks and improved social support between the women and the providers of health services delivery (Manandhar et al., 2004).

People can therefore become involved in a meaningful way by taking part in decision making. The role of the Practitioner shifts to being an 'enabler', gaining the trust of and establishing common ground with their clients. This is crucial to the process of empowerment. Whilst Practitioners cannot be expected to have an influence on transforming power relationships across all sectors and at all levels of their everyday work there are two areas in which they do have an important role:

1. Practitioners are involved in influencing policies and practices that affect health, from national 'down' to the community level, for example, through their 'expert' power in meetings, technical advisory groups and committees. In order to influence policy and practice, Practitioners need to have a better understanding of the meaning of power and how their relationships with different clients are understood and appropriately acted upon by the profession. This is explained in Chapter 2.
2. In most democratic countries, the process of collective action is used to influence social and political changes through public, economic and regulatory policies. These changes are achieved through the legitimate action of individuals who use their decision-making power, for example, to vote. Practitioners, involved in their day-to-day work with individuals and groups, can help their clients to use their power-over decisions to have a greater influence over factors that influence their lives, including their health. To be more empowering in their work Practitioners need to have a clear understanding about the influence that they can have on the process of community empowerment when working with individuals, groups and communities and this is discussed in Chapters 4, 5 and 6.

In practice, an empowering approach to public health involves helping individuals, and the groups and communities in which people participate, to gain power. It also means helping individuals to increase their control over the decisions which influence their lives and their participation in groups and organisations that share their concerns. Participation in interest groups and organisations is the first step for many individuals towards community action. In turn, a collective and more organised context, such as community-based organisations, provide the Practitioner with the opportunity to more effectively help others to increase their knowledge, skills and competencies.

■ The evolution of empowerment in public health practice

Empowerment is defined here as a process by which people are able to gain or seize power (control) over decisions and resources that influence their lives. In the United Kingdom, for example, this concept evolved in public health as an important ideology in the mid-nineteenth century. The political liberalism of the Victorian period led to the creation of many pressure groups, such as the Health of Towns Association, with a concern for equity and social justice. These pressure groups, with the assistance of key public health reformers such as Edwin Chadwick were active in mobilising the middle classes who in turn had an influence on the press and on the government. This is called the 'sanitation phase' and was a period that through both influential reformers and collective action resulted in the government passing key public health legislation such as the 1833 Factories Act and the 1848 Public Health Act (Baggott, 2000). However, these actions were also influenced by the desire of the government to reduce their own responsibilities and to improve the efficiency of the nation's workforce. Public health reform was as much due to the discourse of economic production as it was to the discourse of empowerment and to good governance. During the second phase, occupying the first half of the twentieth century, the growing status of the medical profession added to the political influence of the public health lobby. Consequently, the emphasis was on a public health dominated by a bio-medical model and a focus on the absence of disease and illness.

It was not until the 1960s and 1970s that empowerment became part of the discourse stemming from a growing body of 'new knowledge' that sought to challenge conventional thinking. Within public health, the discourse also broadened from the bio-medical model to include a behavioural and lifestyle component. The main reasons for this change in thinking were an increase in the role of chronic degenerative diseases such as heart disease as the leading causes of morbidity and mortality. These chronic diseases involve the interplay of different factors or determinants over time such as smoking, lack of exercise and a poor diet and have become synonymous with a healthy lifestyle. However public health, at the time closely associated with health education, placed an emphasis on the responsibility of the individual and on a 'victim-blaming' philosophy rather than on collective action and social equity. Internationally, the need for social justice in the challenge to improve health was increasingly recognised and became the subject of professional discourse, for example, the 30th World Health Assembly, held in Geneva in May 1977, which set the target of health for all by the year 2000. The following year, an international conference on primary health care in Alma Ata in the former USSR endorsed this and strongly affirmed the WHO's positive definition of health (World Health Organisation, 1986), noting that it was a fundamental human right. The Alma Ata Declaration of 1978 recognised that the gross inequalities in the health status between and within countries was unacceptable and identified primary health care as the key to attaining health for all by the year 2000. The Declaration recognised that people must be actively involved in the process of development and states: 'The people have the right and duty to participate individually and collectively in the planning and implementation of their health care' (World Health Organisation, 1978, p. 1). The declaration goes beyond participation to imply that empowerment is a necessary component to primary health care and public health.

The Alma Ata Declaration does not use the term empowerment but many of its points imply involvement by individuals and the community. This is in part a reflection of the discourse in the early 1970s when the concept of empowerment had not become fully legitimised. The concept of community participation was viewed as a means to target people as beneficiaries of development by involving them in the process. The discourse argued that participation would allow local knowledge and needs to be incorporated into a programme and would give the people more control in decision making. In practice, this depends on the power relationships between Practitioners and their clients. If Practitioners use their power to take a paternalistic stance, it can lead to community coercion over programme planning and implementation by an outside agent.

Since the early 1980s there has been a shift within public health towards empowerment and community participation embodied in the socio-environmental approach (Robertson and Minkler, 1994). This shift was guided by key strategic documents, such as the Ottawa Charter for Health Promotion (WHO, 1986) and the Bangkok Charter for Health Promotion in a Globalised World (WHO, 2005), but was also due to other contributory factors of a social nature. One of these factors was an increased awareness of growing inequalities in health status between different social groups and the narrowness of the focus on individual behaviour that ignored the psychosocial and physical environments, community and culture. It was recognised that the individualistic nature of public health education campaigns did not recognise the social and environmental contexts in which personal behaviours are embedded and which were important health determinants. Another significant factor was the maturing of many pressure groups and social movements such as the environment movements, the gay rights and Health Social Movements, who challenged the notion of the medical and behavioural approaches to health and raised concerns for social justice and environmental sustainability (Freeman, 1983). The role of Health Social Movements in public health is discussed in Chapter 5.

■ Power and public health practice

□ A bureaucratic setting

The public health profession provides a network of Practitioners that dispense 'expert' advice and services largely through bureaucratic settings. A bureaucratic setting consists of a number of distinctive positions of control (power) with specialist duties that are usually formally defined. The officials who hold these positions of power are recruited according to specific rules and their employment is usually based on a system of salaries. Power is hierarchically top-down and the official is expected to act in accordance with, and without challenging, the instructions descending from their superiors (Turner, 1995). Examples of highly bureaucratic and hierarchical public health organisations include government departments and hospitals. Positioning oneself within the hierarchy of a bureaucratic setting provides a professional legitimacy and status. This is achieved not necessarily because that person has particular expertise but because the institutionalisation of the position creates the idea that she/he is an expert. Within bureaucratic settings Practitioners can however be attributed more occupational autonomy over the process by which a particular service is delivered, for example, individual nurses who did not have to seek approval for every action were found to act more autonomously than on a closely managed ward (Kendall, 1998, p. 25).

☐   The hegemony of the medical profession

The rise of the medical profession has been successful in maintaining its position of dominance within the public health bureaucratic hierarchy by controlling access to health care delivery. This has been termed the 'hegemony of the medical profession'. Hegemonic power is a form that is invisible and internalised such that it is structured into our everyday lives and taken for granted (Foucault, 1979) and is discussed in more detail in Chapter 2. The medical profession has formed itself as a powerful professional pressure group both as a collective work force and through key associations, for example in the UK, the British Medical Association and the Royal Colleges. The medical profession, although not a complete monopoly because of the growth of other health professions, has been granted considerable control to maintain self-regulation and clinical autonomy in their work. In fact, the dominance of the medical profession has been blamed for the historical sub-ordination of the nursing profession and a key challenge to nurse empowerment (Kendall, 1998, p. 33). Much of the power held by the medical profession is also supported by the public who expect confidentiality in the special relationship that they hold with their doctor. The medical profession is also dependent on various alliances with other health professionals, the government, the private sector, science and activists in civil society. It has been careful to create an alignment between both professional and public interests, for example, in regard to the under-resourcing of the UK National Health Service, long waiting times for treatment and the unacceptable demands placed on hospital staff. This professional dom-inance has also been paralleled with an increase in the legitimacy of medical knowledge, urbanisation, the expansion of health insurance and the growth of bureaucratic settings such as hospitals as centres for 'professional excellence' (Turner, 1995). However, there have been challenges to the expert wisdom of medicine from, for example, through the Health Social Movements and lay epidemiology.

☐   Lay epidemiology

Lay epidemiology is a term that has been widely used to describe the processes by which people in their everyday life understand and interpret health risks (Allmark and Tod, 2006). To reach conclusions about the risks to their health they access information from a variety of sources including the mass media, the internet, friends and family. Lay epidemiology presents a challenge to the accepted 'wis-dom' of public health in at least two ways:

1. People through reaching their conclusions do not necessarily accept health messages. People have recognised that some health messages are 'half truths' and this is further confused by the changing of some messaging, for example, in regard to safe limits for alcohol consumption. The prevention paradox is that targeting the behaviour of the majority who are at a low to medium risk has little effect at the individual level. For example, reducing dietary fat

consumption for the whole population would reduce coronary heart disease but it is difficult to change the behaviour of those whose risk is only low to medium. Practitioners have therefore chosen to use simple messaging that does not tell the whole truth by exaggerating the risks of a particular behaviour or the benefits of changing that behaviour. A reliance on health education approaches has led to mistrust in the public and when people feel that the risk does not apply to them, a rejection of the advice (Hunt and Emslie, 2001; Rose, 1985);

2. People also have cultural and personal values that undermine the meaning of health messages, for example, a person can choose not to give up smoking simply because it may be damaging to their health when they believe that the benefits of smoking such as pleasure and reducing stress, outweigh the risk. People can view any particular health behaviour in at least three ways: 1. It is bad because it is poisonous 2. It is bad but desirable such as drinking alcohol 3. It is bad in some ways but good in others such as smoking. People's perception of risk therefore depends on their circumstances, culture and values and an 'all things considered' approach is taken. This is in contrast to traditional epidemiology which is purely empirical (Allmark and Tod, 2006).

Lay epidemiology is the basis for many empowerment approaches. As I discuss in Chapter 3, the empowerment element of a programme is based on the concerns of the community. Communities are influenced by the information that they receive from the many, and sometimes conflicting, sources and that they feel can place them at risk. For example, in the UK public concerns were raised about the MMR (Measles, Mumps and Rubella) vaccine. The public health authorities saw this as an effective option with few side effects. However, following media reports of conflicting scientific evidence the public became increasingly concerned that the vaccine could lead to bowel disease and autism. These concerns were further confounded by past distrust between the authorities and the public over the handling of 'mad cow disease' (Bovine Spongiform Encephalopathy or BSE) and conflicting evidence on the benefits of screening, for example, the benefits of mammography (Smith, 2002). Attempts to coerce or manipulate the public can mean that lay epidemiology becomes a pathway for the community-based actions of a dissatisfied public that lead to collective empowerment.

The public health view has historically been the unquestioned truth. But in an increasingly postmodern world there is no 'truth' whether defined by public health or any other experts. There are different opinions based on different views and theories none of which hold an absolute truth. Lay epidemiology poses a threat to public health because it challenges the accepted wisdom which then is no longer the dominant perspective. Of course, the means of governing people, governmentality, is dependent on 'expert' systems of knowledge, science and empirical truths. This is the means by which to regulate how professionals are empowered to control health care, knowledge and a variety of social problems that do not necessarily fall within the biomedical sphere. The authority structures in regard to health are part of the power-over that the state has on society (Brown and Zavestoski, 2004).

The public is open to rational discussion and Practitioners are right to engage with communities to offer advice that is based on sound scientific evidence. Public health experts have therefore played an important mediating role between those in authority and individuals and social organisations by helping to shape their daily conduct through rationality and self-regulation. Public health provides a measure of the well-being of populations, documenting and establishing trends based on its 'expert' and 'legitimate' power. This sets standards of 'normality' that can be compared in relation to other population groups. In this way, public health practice can build upon political concerns and create issues that they show can be overcome by using their 'expert' knowledge and power. Public health becomes a coercive and manipulative way to influence the way people think and act (Lupton, 1995). This is not always intentional on the part of the Practitioners who face the challenge of meeting targets based on empirical, bio-medical outcomes and which the public may not be ready or willing to engage with. The danger is that public health can present an illusion of greater individual and collective choice whilst acting to hide an agenda that intends to control others to do what we as professionals want them to do, even against their will. Public health then becomes the very opposite of an empowering practice.

☐   Using professional power in public health

If it is true that public health is a bureaucratic activity, carried out by or within governmental organisations or government funded agencies, it is also true that many of these organisations remain chained to traditional ways of thinking and acting, ways which inhibit the effective inclusion of empowering approaches. Various studies of both government and NGO agencies have found that the concept of empowerment used in policy and in practice are often quite different. Despite the intent to 'empower' communities, the organisations and their staff tended to retain control over programming rather than to relinquish power to others. The agencies operated within a contradiction between discourse and practice; many Practitioners continued to exert power-over the community through top-down programming whilst at the same time using an emancipatory discourse (Grace, 1991; Turbyne, 1996).

To build a more empowering practice, public health must redress the constraints placed on the profession by its bureaucratic nature and by other associated professional health groups who do not share an ideology of empowerment. As I discuss in Chapter 2, before Practitioners can empower others they must first be themselves empowered and understand the sources of their own power. This has been argued in the context of a nursing profession that cannot be empowered unless individual nurses themselves are empowered and can be extended to a bureaucratic work setting such as a hospital; a community of both patients and staff. Both must be empowered and this includes feeling valued and having the resources, skills and knowledge to empower others (Kendall, 1998, p. 14).

But governments and the bureaucracies that they create, at least in democratic countries, are not monolithic entities. Not only are there often contradictions between the policies and actions of different government agencies but different Practitioners with differing ideas often exist and work together. Practitioners working in large bureaucratic settings can find their professional autonomy being undermined by the hierarchical structure of rules and lines of control. Professional groups can also become fragmented into sub-groups or else their power base is encroached upon by para-professional groups. These circumstances actually present opportunities for an empowering practice to develop within even the largest, most rigid bureaucracies. To take advantage of these opportunities public health agencies must understand how to address imbalances in the power relationships in their structures and systems at all levels from the top tiers of policy and planning 'down' to the people working at the interface with the community. It is precisely this type of a fundamental issue that must be addressed if Practitioners are to engage an empowering approach in their daily practice. In a professional context the key question is: Do Practitioners *really* want to help to empower people or to simply change their behaviour? The latter has traditionally been the most popular choice and the difference between an empowering approach and a coercive approach has been in the method used. If the method is directive, top-down and controlled by an outside agent it is less likely to be empowering. If it facilitates a process of problem identification and actions based on the concerns of the individual or community and uses capacity building strategies it will have a much better chance of being empowering. Practitioners must make the decision to empower themselves, to gain the necessary skills and knowledge, if they are really committed to an approach that will empower others. Empowerment approaches are also dependent on funding and on there being a political will to implement them. This may be problematic when the goal of the people who are involved in community empowerment is to bring about a change in the political order and to challenge the very agencies that fund and support their continuation. This can create an untrusting relationship between formal agencies and the community. It is a power relationship that must be equalised and which is a central theme of this book.

■ Public health practice and the interpretation of health

The multiplicity of meanings assigned to public health is also a function of the multiplicity of meanings assigned to our understandings of health. In particular, it is useful to consider the distinction between official understandings, those used by public health professionals, and lay understandings, the more popular perceptions held by those who are usually the recipients of health interventions, the public. Practitioners have largely used official interpretations because these are easier to define and measure, rather than lay interpretations of health, which are subjective, being based on the experiences of the individual. In particular, the biomedical interpretation of health has established itself as the most dominant official interpretation. It is the medical profession, which has been the champion of this model of health, based on the absence of disease and illness, and upon which other health professions have modeled themselves including the field of public health and nursing.

The bio-medical model evolved as a result of scientific discoveries and technological advances in the eighteenth and nineteenth centuries and this led to a greater understanding of the structure and functioning of the human body. As knowledge and understanding about the functioning of the human body increased, health took on an increasingly mechanistic meaning. The body was viewed as a machine that needed to be fixed. A professional split between the body and mind developed, the body and its physical illness was the responsibility of physicians while psychologists and psychiatrists looked after the psyche and its illnesses. However, the focus remained on the external causes of ill health and was reinforced by the constant threat of disease and death from epidemics such as polio and scarlet fever (Laverack, 2005).

Peter Aggleton (1991), a commentator on public health issues, divides the official interpretations of health into two main types: those, which define health negatively, and those, which adopt a more positive stance. There are two main ways of viewing health negatively. The first equates with the absence of disease or bodily abnormality, the second with the absence of illness or the feelings of anxiety, pain or distress that may or may not accompany the disease. Aggleton points to the importance of recognising that some people may be diseased without knowing it. People are unaware of their illnesses until they start to suffer pain and discomfort, when the person is said to be ill. Negative definitions of health emphasise the absence of disease or illness and are the basis for the medical model. A number of problems have been raised concerning the negative definition of health. In particular, the notion of pathology implies that certain universal 'norms' exist against which an individual can be assessed when making a judgement as to whether or not they are healthy. This assumes that such standards actually exist in human anatomy and physiology.

Positive interpretations of health have also been widely used by health professionals. The first modern positive definition of health came in 1948 when the World Health Organisation (WHO) stated that health was 'a state of complete physical, social and mental well-being, and not merely the absence of disease or infirmity' (Jackson et al., 1989). Physical well-being is concerned with concepts such as the proper functioning of the body, biological normality, physical fitness and capacity to perform tasks. Social well-being includes interpersonal relationships as well as wider social issues such as marital satisfaction, employability and community involvement. The role of relations, the family and status at work are important to a person's social well-being. Mental well-being involves concepts such as self-efficacy, subjective well-being and social inclusion and is the ability of people to adapt to their environment and the society in which they function. The WHO definition has become one of the most influential and commonly used in public health and for that reason its origins, which are set in the context of empowerment, are worthwhile exploring in Box 1.1.

The WHO definition of health, as an ideal state of physical, social and mental well-being has been criticised for not taking other dimensions of health into

Box 1.1 The Origins of the WHO Definition of 'Health'

The WHO definition was written soon after the Second World War by an official who had spent his time working in the Resistance. He had come to this definition from his experience and explained that he had never felt healthier than during that terrible period: for he daily worked for goals about which he cared passionately, he was certain that should he be killed in his dangerous work, his family would be cared for by the network of Resistance workers. It was under these circumstances that he felt most healthy, most alive. The definition of health was developed by a person who was passionately involved with others to change social and political structures. In other words, they were involved in taking control over those things which affect their lives and by doing so empowered themselves and improved their own health and well-being as well as that of others with whom they associated (Jackson et al., 1989).

account, namely the emotional and spiritual aspects of health (Ewles and Simnett, 2003). The definition has also been criticised for viewing health as a state or product rather than as a dynamic relationship, a capacity, a potential or a process and does not clarify how to define or measure its components.

The way in which people interpret the meaning of their own health is a personal and sometimes unique experience. Health is a subjective concept and its interpretation is relative to the environment and culture in which people find themselves. Health can mean different things to different people. Many people define health in functional terms by their ability to carry out certain roles and responsibilities rather than the absence of disease. People may be willing to bear the discomfort and pain of an illness because it does not outweigh the inconvenience, loss of control or financial cost of having the condition treated (Laverack, 2005).

This subjective view of health raises the issue of radical relativism which maintains that the only 'true' reality is the unique experience of the individual. Whilst it is important to understand individual feelings and experiences about health there may be others that are common to particular groups. Inter-subjectivity is a concept used to overcome the limitations of radical relativism. It claims that any given person's understanding of the world is unique but because it is constructed from a field of more or less common social meanings and experiences, communication between people is possible. In other words, the meanings we create of our own experiences, for example of health, overlap sufficiently so that we can communicate and share these with others. The importance of personal interpretations of health is becoming increasing well recognised, for example, the link between individual control and health has been demonstrated in several studies (Brunner, 1996; Everson et al., 1997). Everson et al. (1997) undertook a study of Finnish middle-aged white males and concluded that stress induced from job demands and feelings of a lack of control was the strongest predictor of arterial heart disease. A review of heart health inequalities in Canada found that people who experience low income, less control in their lives and at work and who had a poor education are more likely to experience morbidity and mortality. In other words, the higher one's position in the workplace or society, one's power (control), wealth and status, the better one's health and sense of self-esteem (Labonte, 1993).

Self-esteem is actually a social phenomenon and not an individual creation. A person's self-regard and sense of coherence is not grounded in 'the self', but in relation to friends, family, colleagues, the communities and settings in which they live and work. Social support is therefore also generally accepted as having a beneficial effect on health, both at home or in the community; for example, by sharing problems people are better able to cope with stressful events. Social support is connected to other similar overlapping concepts such as social capital, social inclusiveness, social exclusiveness and social cohesion. These concepts fundamentally address a sense of connection to a 'community' and the involvement and trust between its members manifested through customs, rituals and traditional groupings such as weddings.

Official definitions of health can differ significantly from lay definitions but both are ideal types and in practice coexist and inform one another. Practitioners have embraced a discourse that uses an official definition that goes beyond health care and lifestyle to feelings of well-being. Health is considered to be a means to an end that can be expressed in functional terms as a resource which permits people to lead an individually, socially and economically productive life. However, in practice, public health programming has increasingly been concerned with accountability to funders, effectiveness and value for money (Boutilier, 1993). Budgetary constraints, competition for funding and priorities for health have also had a strong influence on the way in which health has been interpreted. The public health profession has taken the pragmatic view that whatever interpretation of health is used it must be measurable and accountable, otherwise programmes employing its ideology and strategies will be in jeopardy of being unable to justify their economic and quantifiable effectiveness. This being the case, the measurement of health has focused on the bio-medical approach that is concerned with demonstrating a relationship between a health status measure and a behaviour such as smoking or a condition such as mortality. The boundaries for public health practice and discourse have consequently been defined by the interpretations of illness and disease rather than by the way in which most people generally view their own health.

Next in Chapter 2, I move the reader into the territory of how power, as a concept, is central to public health practice; what power looks like; what the means to attaining power is and how Practitioners can act to transform personal and social power relationships at the individual, group and community levels.

Chapter 2

Power and empowerment

Power and empowerment are central to public health and yet many Practitioners still have a superficial understanding of their different meanings. In particular, how these two concepts can be applied as a part of their everyday work. In public health today there exists a contradiction between professional discourse and practice: many Practitioners continue to exert power-over their clients through 'top-down' programming and controlling working practices whilst at the same time using an emancipatory ideology and language. Plainly put, many Practitioners do not have a clear understanding of how the empowerment of individuals, groups and communities can be practically accommodated within public health practice. However, the situation is more complicated than this and to simply blame the Practitioner would be to underestimate the important role that they can have in empowering their clients. For public health to use an empowering approach, its members need to understand how power is an integral part of the relationship between Practitioners and their clients, and how they can transform this relationship to help others gain more power.

■ What is power?

The most common interpretation of power used in the literature is in the form of one person or group having power-over and mastery of others or 'the capacity of some persons to produce intended and foreseen effects on others' (Wrong, 1988, p. 2). The anthropologist, Richard Adams (1977) further discusses the idea that power can be a social phenomenon, one that can be vested in both individuals and social groups. As social organisations and communities develop, they are better able to identify and control the basis of their power. The concept of power can be viewed as both a limited, finite entity (zero-sum) and as an expanding, infinite entity (non-zero-sum). These are important distinctions for public health practice that I will discuss later in this chapter.

To exercise choice is the simplest form of power. This may involve the trivial health choices of everyday life such as which brand of toothpaste to buy or the more critical choices such as whether or not to stop smoking. Practitioners should recognise that the rhetoric of choice can become an excuse for health professionals to avoid difficult issues and to transfer blame. The trivial choices should not cloud the more critical issues where the powerless have no choice, for example, promoting an active lifestyle when poor people cannot afford, do not have the time or a supportive environment in which to do more exercise. Box 2.1 provides

Box 2.1   The Safer Parks Scheme in New Zealand

The Safer Parks Scheme in Christchurch, New Zealand was started in 1993 by the City Council following many complaints about crime, including sexual attacks, in public parks. These open areas provided facilities for people to do more exercise such as walking and cycling which were not being used because of the fear of attack. The Safer Parks Scheme invested in employing more park wardens and honorary rangers to patrol the areas, installing cycle ways and play equipment for children to make access easier. The Scheme encouraged public participation through its 'adopt a park' initiative and recruited volunteers to help to raise sponsorship money, to provide preservation and protection work and to report any problems that they encountered in the parks. The volunteers and the public attended regular meetings to identify problems, solutions and actions and as a result of all these activities park patronage increased (Gee, 2008).

an example how communities got involved in choices about improving lifestyle in the Safer Parks Scheme in Christchurch, New Zealand.

To the extent our personal choices constrain those of others, power becomes an exercise of control. For example, people with the ability to control decisions at the macro (political and economic) level condition and constrain the ability of people to exercise choice at the micro (individual and group) level. People therefore both have control (power)-over others and are constrained and influenced by those that have power-over themselves. To better understand how power can be exercised in both a positive manner (the sharing of control with others) and a negative manner (the use of control to exert influence over others), it is helpful for Practitioners to consider four different variations: 'power-from-within'; 'power-over'; 'power-with'; and powerlessness.

■ Power-from-within

Power-from-within can be described as an experience of 'self ', a personal power or some inner sense of self-knowledge, self-discipline and self-esteem (Labonte, 1996). Power-from-within is also known as individual, personal or psychological empowerment, the means of gaining (a sense of) control over one's life (Rissel, 1994). The goal of psychological empowerment is to increase feelings of value and a sense of personal mastery. Thomas Wartenberg (1990), a writer on the different forms of power, argues that even in the most male-dominated, controlling society, women have power, the power-from-within. Likewise, Western feminist theory claims that although women are not socially dominant, they do have special skills and inner strengths that have enabled them to act in invaluable ways. Once one has accepted this, Wartenberg's (1990, p. 188) argument that 'the seemingly contradictory claim that women both have and lack power in a male dominated society' can be seen to contain an important insight because it makes power a decentred notion. Individuals can become more powerful from within and do not necessarily have to accumulate money, status or authority. However the individualisation of this concept can lead to public health approaches that aim to increase the notion of 'self', for example in assertiveness classes, ignoring how another form of power, power-over, can constrain experiences of control in the 'real world' (Laverack, 2004).

■ Power-over

Power-over describes social relationships in which one party is made to do what another party wishes them to, despite their resistance and even if it may not be in their best interests. Starhawk (1990, p. 9) describes power-over in its rawest form as 'the power of the prison guard, of the gun, power that is ultimately backed by force'. However the exercise of power-over does not always have to be negative, for example, legislation to control the spread of diseases through quarantine or to impose fines for unhygienic behaviour such as for food handlers not washing their hands, are considered as 'healthy' power-over.

Power-over can take different forms depending on how it is used to exert control or to affect the actions of others: dominance, or the direct power to control people's choices, usually by force or its threat; hegemony, or the ability of a dominant group to control the actions and behaviours of others by intense persuasion and exploit-ation, or the indirect power to control people's choices through economic relations, in which those who control capital also have control over those who do not (Wrong, 1988). Speer and Hughley (1995) discuss three instruments of material power-over in relation to its oppressive use in Appalachian communities in North America. The first instrument of power is manifested through superior bargaining resources that can be used to reward and punish. Therefore, those with the greatest resources have the greatest power. A second instrument of power is the ability to construct barriers to participation or eliminate barriers to participation through setting agendas and defining issues. Thus by controlling access to decision-making processes, the topics and timing of discussion those with power can effectively limit participation and per-spectives in public debate. The third instrument of power is a force that influences or shapes shared consciousness through the control of information.

Bertram Raven and Tchia Litman-Adizes (1986) also considered the resources that Practitioners may bring to bear on their client in order to change their beliefs, attitudes and behaviours. These are identified as six bases of power-over: coer-cion; reward; legitimacy; expertise; reference and information. To put the six bases of power-over into context I now provide a brief example for each in regard to breast feeding although there are many other examples of the six bases of power in public health practice:

1. In **coercive power**, the Practitioner may bring about negative consequences or punishment for the woman if she does not comply, for example, using disapproving language towards her for not breast feeding her child.

2. In **reward power**, the Practitioner may bring about positive consequences for the woman upon compliance, for example by praising her for breast feeding her child and keeping the child clean.

3. **Legitimate power** stems from the woman accepting a social role relationship with the Practitioner, a structural relationship which grants him/her the right to prescribe behaviour for the woman, while the woman accepts an obligation to comply with the requests of the Practitioner. The woman accepts the legitimate professional position of a nurse and listens to and then carries out his/her advice on breast feeding.

4. **Expert power** stems from the woman attributing superior knowledge and ability to the Practitioner, for example, the term 'Doctor knows best' illustrates the expert power relationship between the patient and doctor. The same level of superior knowledge is attributed by the women to the nurse Practitioner.

5. **Referent power** stems from an identification of the woman with the Practitioner, a feeling of communality, similarity, and mutual interest. The woman then gets some satisfaction from believing and complying in a manner consistent with the beliefs, attitudes and behaviours of the Practitioner. This may be based on the gender, social class, ethnicity or empathy shown by a nurse Practitioner toward the breast feeding mother.

6. **Informational power** is based on the explicit information communicated to the woman from the Practitioner, a persuasive communication that will convince the woman that the recommended behaviour is indeed in the woman's best interests (Raven and Litman-Adizes, 1986), for example, advice on appropriate forms of family planning to assist child spacing including breast feeding. Informational power is the form commonly used in health education however it is important to note that the term 'knowledge is power' can be misleading and is not necessarily correct. New knowledge without the means to carry out the prescribed actions can simply lead to people having a greater sense of powerlessness. For example, informing the breast feeding mother to eat healthy foods for the benefit of herself and her child when she cannot afford to buy these products.

◼ Hegemonic power

Hegemonic power is that form of power-over that is invisible and internalised such that it is structured into our everyday lives and taken for granted (Foucault, 1979). To Foucault, a prominent theorist and commentator on power, the only form of resistance to hegemonic power was a concealment of one's life from those in authority and the judgements that it can create. A practical example of this is a single mother living in government-funded housing hiding her sick child from a health visitor (Bloor and McIntosh, 1990) or lowering the toilet seat to avoid suspicion that she was cohabitating with a man. Persons living in conditions of hegemonic power-over, of oppression and exploitation, internalise these conditions as being their personal responsibility. This internalisation increases their own self-blame and decreases their self-esteem. One of the subtle but common ways in which Practitioners participate in hegemonic power is when they continually impose their 'expert' ideas of what are important health problems without listening to what their clients think are the important health concerns.

Piven and Cloward (1977) suggest that in conditions of oppressive forms of power-over and poverty where people have few institutional and material resources, the marginalised cannot rely upon support from the established system. Marginalised groups must then use the only significant resource they have, the capacity to cause trouble. The tactics used are protests, riots, demonstrations, strikes taking legal action, funding an aggressive publicity campaign or actively lobbying people in positions of power. Table 2.1 provides further examples of this type of direct disruptive action. The disruption, public support and the reaction of those in authority become the basis for greater political influence. This is a limited option

Table 2.1 Direct actions towards empowerment

	Non-violent actions	Peaceful civil protests and demonstrations such as 'sit-ins'.
Direct Actions		Refusal to pay taxes or bills.
		Infiltrate a meeting such as one being held by shareholders.
		Take part in a boycott or strike action.
		Create a media event such as climbing a public building to deploy a banner.
		Engage in an aggressive publicity campaign.
		Instigate legal action against someone else.
	Violent actions (physical action against people or property)	Hack into another computer ('Hacktivism') to obtain information or to insert a virus package.
		Physically alter something to prevent action such as 'spiking' trees with metal pins.
		Place oneself in a position of manufactured vulnerability to prevent action such as building and occupying a tunnel under a road or a tree house, squatting in a house detailed for demolition.
		Take part in a riot or revolt with the intention to carry out physical damage on property or persons.

but historically it has given rise to examples of dramatic change, for example, the collective action of lower-class tenants in the United States of America in regard to poor housing in the middle years of the twentieth century. The crux of Piven and Cloward's argument is to maximise these occasions and to push for full concessions in return for a cease to disruption. It can be the most effective means of utilising the limited resources available to people living under non-supportive, repressive social and political conditions.

■ Power-with

Power-with describes a different set of social relationships, in which power-over is used carefully and deliberately to increase other people's power, rather than to dominate or exploit them. Power-over transforms to power-with only when it has effectively reached its end, when the submissive person in the relationship has accrued enough power-from-within to exercise his or her own choices and decisions. The person with the power-over chooses not to command or exert control, but to suggest and to begin a discussion that will increase the other's level of control. The Practitioner offers advice to their clients in the identification and resolution of problems to help develop their power-from-within and their competence. The transformative use of power-over also demands a great deal of self-vigilance and self-discipline by all persons in the relationship, but in particular by the initially more dominant person, the Practitioner. If not, the relationship can remain as power-over, for example, using the different instruments of social power discussed above by Raven and Litman-Adizes (1986): referent power or mentoring that does not try to come to completion can become charismatic authority or 'guruisation'; and legitimate or expert power that does not acknowledge that others in the relationship may have their own expertise can lead to a patronising inducement of dependency.

An example of the delicate balance of the transformative use of power-over at an individual level can be illustrated in the doctor-patient relationship. This professional relationship has traditionally been paternalistic and unequal where all competence and expertise is often considered to belong to one party, the person with the power-over or the doctor. The doctor (after an examination) tells the patient what their medical problem is and prescribes a treatment for it. The patient voluntarily surrenders to the unspoken claim of medical (expert) power, for example, the phrase 'Doctor knows best' epitomises this situation. The doctor has control over the knowledge even though that knowledge concerns the patient's own body. The attributes of health are viewed as an individual 'case' and the diagnosis is made on the basis of the medical model (the presence or absence of disease or illness) that serves to protect the legitimate and expert bases of power held by the doctor. However, in the health system, the power-over relationship does not stop at diagnosis because the doctor often also controls the admission and discharge, choice of treatment, referral and care of the patient.

A power-with doctor-patient relationship would be more equal. One in which the doctor uses their knowledge to allow the patient to make informed decisions

Box 2.2 The Patient-centered Clinical Method

1. The illness and the patient's experience of being ill are explored at the same time;
2. Understanding the person as a whole places the illness into context by considering how does the illness affect the person?, how does the person interact with their immediate environment?, How does the wider environment influence this interaction?;
3. The patient and doctor reach a mutual understanding on the nature of the illness its causes and its goals for management, and who is responsible for what;
4. The desirability and applicability to undertake broader health promoting and illness prevention tasks, for example, providing the patient with information or skills about how he/she themselves can dress a wound at home;
5. Gaining a better understanding of the patient-doctor relationship in order to enhance it, for example, placing a value on the contribution being made by both sides and forming a 'partnership' to address the illness rather than a traditional paternalistic approach;
6. Making a realistic assessment of what can be done to help the patient given, for example, constraints in understanding, time and skill level (Stewart, Brown, Weston et al., 2003).

about their treatment and recovery. In effect, the patient is placed at the centre of the issue requiring the doctor to gain as much information as possible from their experience rather than what the doctor should achieve in the consultation. The patient-centered clinical method applies the principles of a power-with Practitioner-patient relationship and the six interactive components of this approach are provided in Box 2.2.

Giving the client more control over decisions that influence their health, well-being and recovery can occur as part of home-based treatment, care for the dying (palliative care) and chronic conditions. Box 2.3 provides an example of how giving a patient more control over decisions related to home-based care can demonstrate real benefits.

■ Zero-sum and non-zero-sum forms of power

Zero-sum power exists when one can only possess x amount of power to the extent that someone else has the absence of an equivalent amount. It is therefore a 'win/lose' situation. My power-over you, plus your absence of that power, equals zero (thus the term, 'zero-sum'). I win and you lose. For you to gain power, you must seize it from me. If you can, you win and I lose. Power is used as leverage to

Box 2.3 Empowering Individual Patients for Home-based Care

Giving the client more control over decisions can have real benefits as demonstrated in one study (Bassett and Prapavessis, 2007) on physical therapy for ankle sprains. The study showed that the home-based groups had similar outcome scores for post-treatment ankle function, adherence and motivation to a standard physical therapy intervention. However, the home-based group had significantly better attendance at clinic appointments and a better physical therapy completion rate. Patients were helped to set goals and to develop personal action plans to complete the therapy as well as education and skills training on the treatment such as strapping techniques. The patients had more control and were better informed about their recovery and this sharing of the power (knowledge, skills) by the Practitioner was a form of power-with which led to a viable home-based option for the clients. Self-care can be a complicated issue that is not appropriate for all situations or people but under the right conditions, as this study showed, can offer the Practitioner the opportunity to work in a more empowering way.

raise the position of one person or group, while simultaneously lowering it for another person or group. However, at any one time there will be only so much leverage (wealth, control, resources) possessed within a society. This distribution and the decision-making authority that goes with it is zero-sum. At the same time, there are dominant forms of status or privilege, such as class, gender, education and ethnic background that tend to structure power-over relations in most social situations. The role of the Practitioner in this zero-sum construction of power is to assist individuals, groups and communities to gain power (meaning here more control over resources or decision making that influence their health and lives), from other individuals, groups and communities. Practitioners, in the course of their work, may find it unavoidable to help some people but not others. Public health policy sometimes places such a requirement on Practitioners to work with specific groups such as the poor, the homeless or the 'unhealthy'. It is based on the interpretation of power as being resource dependent and reliant on some type of a material product. It essentially ignores that power may also be a property of social relations including the relationship one has with oneself (power-from-within) (Clegg, 1989). Zakus and Lysack (1998) provide an interesting point of view in relation to a zero-sum construction of power which they argue increases competition and a lack of community cohesion. They suggest that 'community empowerment' is a contradiction in terms and that by empowering some at the expense of others, Practitioners are actually breaking down the ties that hold a community together. Some gain more control but the community as a whole starts to disintegrate. Competing groups within a community can be willing to put aside their differences to organise and mobilise themselves around shared concerns. This then creates a 'community of interest' with which the Practitioner can work to help them to gain power.

There is another important concept of power, one that is regarded not as fixed and finite, but as infinite and expanding. These 'non-zero-sum' forms of power are 'win/win', since they are based on the idea that if any one person or group gains, everyone else also gains. Trust, caring and other aspects of our social relationships with one another are examples of non-zero-sum power. To be more empowering in their work, Practitioners should gravitate towards the non-zero-sum formulation. Power is no longer seen as a finite commodity, such as wealth, or as the comparative status and authority that this might confer. Rather, non-zero-sum power takes the form of relationship behaviours based on respect, generosity, service to others, a free flow of information and the commitment to the ethics of caring and justice. The role of the Practitioner in this construction of power is to use these attributes to engender them in others and to transfer power by encouraging individuals to access information for themselves, in part by providing better access to resources (Laverack, 2004).

In practice, public health simultaneously involves zero-sum and non-zero-sum formulations of power. Power cannot be given but communities can be enabled by Practitioners to gain or seize power from others. Practitioners must first identify their own power bases and then through the professional-client relationship to share these to enable others to gain control over the influences on their lives and health. Practitioners need to know both how to use their own power to help themselves into a position of more control and how to help others to gain power. To help them, Practitioners generally do have more power or a stronger power base than their clients, for example, their education level and professional training, higher incomes, expert status and social class, access to information and resources, influence over decision makers, familiarity with systems of bureaucracy and control over budget allocations.

■ Powerlessness

Powerlessness, or the absence of power, whether imagined or real, is an individual concept with the expectancy that the behaviour of a person cannot determine the outcomes they seek. It combines an attitude of self-blame, a sense of generalised distrust, a feeling of alienation from resources for social influence, an experience of disenfranchisement and economic vulnerability, and a sense of hopelessness in gaining social and political influence (Kieffer, 1984). The process by which people may perceive themselves as being powerless is described in Box 2.4.

Michael Lerner (1986), a political scientist and psychotherapist, argues that a similar phenomenon occurs with persons living in risk conditions. He named this process 'surplus powerlessness', a surplus created by, but distinct from, external or objective conditions of powerlessness. In surplus powerlessness individuals internalise their objective or external powerlessness and create a potent psychological barrier to empowering action. They do not even engage in activities that meet their real needs. They begin to accept aspects of their world that are self-destructive to their own health and well-being, thinking that these are unalterable features of

Box 2.4 Experiencing Powerlessness

The process by which people may perceive themselves as being powerless can begin when individuals and groups living in risk conditions or who experience inequalities in health (poor housing, unemployment, insanitary conditions) feel distress with the unfairness of their situation (their low status on some hierarchy of power or authority, indicated in part by wealth). These people then internalise this feeling of unfairness as aspects of their own 'badness' or 'failure'. This internalisation adds to their distress, if not also to their loss of meaning and purpose, with measurable effects on their bodies such as hypertension (Labonte, 1998). The powerless often experience little leverage on the events and conditions that impinge on their existence, either directly or through access to resources, information and facilities. This situation is made worse, when the dominant social discourse on success is competitiveness, individualism and meritocracy, where people are presumed to succeed or fail purely on the basis of their own initiative or ability (Lerner, 1986). This internalisation of 'badness' leads to what is described as both false consciousness, 'failing to utilize the power that one has and failing to acquire powers that one can acquire' (Morriss, 1987, p. 94), and learned helplessness (Seligman, 1975).

what they take to be 'reality'. Power and powerlessness are relative to that held by others and one has authority or social status by virtue of others not having it. There is a degree of flexibility here, however, since someone may have authority or status in one situation, relative to others, but not in another. For example, a migrant may hold the position of a hereditary chief within his own community, but within his work place in his adopted country, he may have little status. Practitioners therefore need to look for, and work from, areas in powerless peoples' lives in which they are relatively powerful.

▪ Empowerment: the means to attaining power

Empowerment, the means to attaining power, in the broadest sense can be described as 'the process by which disadvantaged people work together to increase control over events that determine their lives' (Werner, 1988, p. 1). Most definitions give the term a similarly positive value and embody the notion that empowerment must come from an individual, group or community. The essence of empowerment is that it cannot be bestowed and must be gained by those who seek it. Those that have power or have access to it, such as Practitioners, and those who want it, such as their clients, must work together to create the conditions necessary to make empowerment possible. In professional practice, this is a mutual role played out by the Practitioner who can facilitate change and the clients who identify and execute the change. However, as discussed above, one must be able to identify one's own power base in order to share it with others. The inability of some Practitioners to identify and activate their power base may account for the act of gaining power being neglected in favour of the act of attempting to help others simply through the delivery of knowledge and other resources.

To provide clarity to the concept of empowerment it is useful to consider three different levels: individual, organisational and community. Christopher Rissel (1994, p. 41) includes a heightened or increased level of psychological (individual) empowerment as a part of community empowerment. He argues that community empowerment includes 'a political action component in which members have actively participated, and the achievement of some redistribution of resources or decision making favourable to the community or group in question'. Barbara Israel and her colleagues (1994) similarly identify psychological and political action as two levels of community empowerment, but include a third, and intermediary level between them, that of organisational empowerment. An empowered organisation is one that is democratically managed, its members share information and control over decisions and are involved in the design, implementation and control of efforts towards goals defined by group consensus.

Haynes and Singh (1993) provide a further model for 'family empowerment' as a social unit within communities which are able to organise themselves into 'advocacy groups' to assist them to gain power. This is a common theme in non-westernised societies where importance is placed on the well-being of social units such as the family rather than on the individual. Public health programmes are very often targeted at the individual, for example, to change behaviour or to increase knowledge. The danger is that this approach can be inappropriately superimposed onto socio-cultural contexts that focus on the family or community unit rather than the individual. The family is the core unit of society in these cultural contexts and the purpose of empowerment is to give people more control at the appropriate level so that they can address their own concerns.

Community empowerment is a synergistic interaction between individual, family and organisational empowerment and broader social and political actions. Community empowerment is both an individual and a group phenomena. It is a dynamic process, involving continual shifts in individual empowerment and changes in power-over relations between different social groups and decision makers in the broader society. Community empowerment is also an outcome and in this form it can vary, for example, as a redistribution of resources (Rappaport, 1984), a decrease in powerlessness or a success in achieving predefined goals (Kieffer, 1984; Rappaport, 1985). But it is most consistently viewed as a process along a continuum representing progressively more organised and broadly-based forms of social and collective action and this is discussed in Chapter 5.

Per-Anders Tengland (2007, p. 205) concludes from a conceptual analysis of collective empowerment that as a means or a process it has applicability for creating freedom or opportunity to improve health. He believes that the logic for using an empowering approach in public health is justified because it is based on well founded theory that has empirical support and that it is ethically or morally sound to do so. He also recognises that many Practitioners do not have the knowledge and skills that are required to undertake an empowering approach and raises the issue of adequate training. Practitioners often work with clients from different cultural backgrounds and they need to have a shared understanding of power and empowerment if they are to use empowering approaches in their everyday work. Training would therefore have to include a better understanding of ourselves as Practitioners, our beliefs and values and to put this into a framework of other social and cultural perceptions of power and empowerment.

■ Social and cultural perceptions of power and empowerment

Many of the definitions of power and empowerment have been developed by psychologists in industrialised countries in the areas of neighbourhood empowerment and community mental health (Rappaport, 1987; Swift and Levin, 1987). But empowerment may hold a very different connotation for people living in different cultural contexts, for example, what might be perceived as empowering by women in an industrialised country may be very different for women in a developing country. This can include the degree of, or expectation of, power-over the events in life such as choosing who to marry, where and with whom to live, what to be employed as, what to wear or even if enough control is permissible, to leave the house alone. Contextual influences such as poverty (economic), social norms (socio-cultural), bureaucratic structures (political), historical and colonial circumstances can also lead to different perceptions of power and empowerment. Next I provide examples of how culture and context can change perceptions of power and empowerment from South and Latin America, Africa and the Pacific.

Sharry Erzinger (1994), a health consultant in Latin America, explains the meaning of empowerment in Ecuador where poverty, religion, superstition and political dominance all function to maintain 'power-over' authority and control in most people's lives. Erzinger points out that in the Spanish language empowerment is not an individual or solitary phenomenon but is connected to the family or community. Maruja Barrig (1990), a community worker in South America, provides an example of how the economic context can also have a positive influence on people's empowerment. Women in Peru, forced by an economic crisis, which led to depressed incomes and unemployment, were placed in a deprived situation and had to empower themselves. Women's community-based organisations helped to establish communal kitchens, to channel relief and to set up self-help groups for the people worst hit by the economic crisis, especially those in the shanty towns. The economic context created desperate conditions, which in turn acted as a 'trigger' for the women to embark on a process of empowerment to bring about action to help themselves and others. The historical context of community action may determine future involvement, set precedents or predetermined assumptions about power and empowerment. A history of resistance between the church in Latin America and the land-owning aristocracy provides the backdrop for a major empowering force through critical reflection. Church activists, inspired by their own theology, rejected the elitist and corrupt practices of the landowners and pioneered resistance movements against those in power. In Latin America, the church continues to promote community action among the poor through co-operative solutions, self-help and participatory approaches (Asthana, 1994). Knowledge of the historical context of the community can help identify potential barriers to community empowerment such as experiences of conflict or feelings of helplessness. Goodman et al. (1998) argue that communities with access to information about their history, verbal or written, have a better chance of affecting change, than those that do not have access. However a historical context of colonialism has been shown to generate an atmosphere in which empowerment is difficult to achieve. Serrano-Garcia (1984) uses Puerto Rico as a case study and argues that an ideology of conservatism and pro-American values has been forced into the culture. The weakening of this ideo-logy was one of the main goals of the Esfuerazo project in order to gain cultural identity, independence and collective empowerment. However, Serrano-Garcia argues that this has only created an illusion of empowerment because newly gained control over a person's life still exists within an oppressive colonial context, which continues to determine the physical and physiological well-being of the population.

Viviene Taylor (1995), a commentator on social welfare and development, in her account of social reconstruction and the transition to democracy in South Africa argues that the inability of those in power (the government) to establish an economic context that absorbed surplus unemployed labour significantly con-tributed to the crisis in that country. The unemployed had no income and many turned to conflict, violence and crime to support themselves and their families and as a result, this led to feelings of powerlessness amongst the population. Gill Gordon (1995), a community development worker, discusses the effects of both the social and economic context on the Krobo people in Ghana, West Africa. To alleviate economic hardship young women have traditionally worked for a few years in the neighbouring country of Ivory Coast in order to purchase essentials and to make enough capital to set themselves up in business. These visits are organised by the older women of the community and it is socially accepted that sexual relationships would contribute to the economic success of these young women. In the mid-1980s young women started to come home with a fatal disease later diagnosed as AIDS. Without better economic alternatives young women continued to follow in the footsteps of their sisters and friends and to continue the cycle of infection. The economic context had led to the need to develop sexual relationships as a means of income but this was maintained because of the social acceptability of this practice. This has had dire consequences for the families of the Krobo people who provide the support and care necessary once the young women develop AIDS.

Laverack, 'Ofanoa, Nosa, Fa'alili and Taufa (2007) undertook a review to iden-tify studies, published papers and grey material regarding the definition of power and empowerment in Pacific Peoples. The predominant perception was of power over an individual or group or as a means whereby people could better themselves within the community through, for example, educational qualifications. In Fiji, Laverack (1998) found that the concept of power was divided between the traditional and cultural authority held by hereditary chiefs and the control that people had in their own homes and at work. The concept of empowerment was not based on an individual level of control but was built around a cultural framework, of for example, returning a favour, supporting other peoples' capacities and working as a team, group or community. The way in which people viewed their role differed from a westernised perception of individual actions and the control over material resources. Kana'iaupuni, (2005) maintains that in a Pacific context knowledge is power, and that power lies in the use of knowledge to advance one understanding of the world as opposed to another. Power is gained when people are given the information or resources that will help them gain knowledge about issues that directly affect them. This process of gaining power does not mean that one person has to give up power in order for another to gain power, but argues that power can be shared between the respective parties provided they had a 'voice'. The concept of gaining/sharing power through knowledge sounds ideal, however for many pacific people the chances of power being passed on in the form of power-over is still more likely than power-from-within. For example, Tonga is a kingdom in which people are ranked on the basis of birth and gender. As well as broad rankings of 'commoner' and 'chief,' everyone within a single family has a hierarchical relationship to one another based on primogeniture and gender (Small, 1999).

Laverack, 'Ofanoa, Nosa, Fa'alili and Taufa (2007) concluded that the implication to public health practice is for more equitable policy to empower Pacific peoples in New Zealand and in particular:

1. To make government support more equitable within Pacific peoples: There has been a tendency in New Zealand health policy to combine the different Pacific peoples together under one ethnic category. Categorising Pacific peoples under one homogeneous group runs the real risk of advantaging some at the expense of others. For example, in a competitive funding environment there should be an equal opportunity policy to access resources that recognises the sometimes subtle differences between Pacific peoples.
2. To build on the specific strengths of Pacific Peoples: To address the broader inequalities in their health, Pacific people have a better chance of success if they can act collectively. It is through collective action that people can increase their access to resources, influence decisions and build support through wider participation. By increasing their membership and resource base, Pacific communities are better able to have an influence on government policy.
3. To assist Pacific people to move toward community empowerment: Government policy can build community support and social interaction by facilitating the many associations, community-based organisations, faith groups and

charitable bodies. Policy that builds community capacity, strengthens alliances between Pacific groups and supports community-empowerment initiatives, are identified as ways forward.

(Laverack and 'Ofanoa et al., 2007, pp. 60–1).

Next, Chapter 3 discusses the tensions that exist in public health and outlines a methodology for 'parallel-tracking' empowerment such that 'top-down' and 'bottom-up' approaches can be accommodated together in the same programme.

Chapter 3

Empowerment and public health programming

■ Introduction

In practice, public health is most commonly implemented as activities set within the context of an intervention, a project or a programme. In this book, I have used the term 'programme' to refer to all these situations. The programme cycle is conventionally managed and monitored by the Practitioner and commonly includes: a period of identification; design; appraisal; approval; implementation; management and evaluation. The technical considerations are documented as an agreement between the different stakeholders in a form that ideally makes sense to everyone involved such as a Memorandum of Understanding or as a logical framework that outlines the aims, objectives, inputs and outputs and other details for the programme.

The way in which public health 'problems' are to be addressed and are defined in a programme is one of the most important issues and can take two main forms: 'top-down' and 'bottom-up'. 'Top-down' describes programmes in which problem identification comes from the top structures in the system down to the community, defined by the outside agent and technical 'experts'. 'Bottom-up' is the reverse in which the community identifies its own problems and communicates these to the top structures. Top-down programming is a manifestation of power-over, in which the Practitioner exercises control of financial and other material resources over the beneficiaries of the programme. It is a form of dominance and authority in which control is exerted through the design, implementation and evaluation of the programme. I intentionally use the terms top-down and bottom-up in this book because they help to illustrate the common power relationship that exists in public health programming: The Practitioner uses their power-over to push down a predefined agenda onto the community with the assumption that power can be given, usually as information or resources.

Top-down and bottom-up approaches are ideal types of best practice and demonstrate the important differences in relation to programme design. In Table 3.1 I show the main differences between the two styles of programme design. In public health programmes the design does not usually include the building of community empowerment as a high level aim. At best, community empowerment is seen as a lower level objective and the main aim of the programme is typically centred on improving health or preventing disease. This can become problematic

29

Table 3.1   The different characteristics of top-down and bottom-up approaches

Characteristic	Top-down approaches	Bottom-up approaches
Role of agents	Outside agents define the issue, develop strategies to resolve the issue, involve the community to assist with solving the issue.	Outside agents act to support the community in the identification of issues which are important and relevant to their lives and enable them to develop strategies to resolve these issues.
Design	Defined short- to medium-term time frame, budget, stakeholder analysis.	Long-term without defined programme time frame.
Objectives	Objectives are determined by outside agent and are usually concerned with changing specific behaviours to reduce disease and improve health.	Community identifies objectives which are negotiated with outside agent. These may be concerned with disease and behaviours, but also with community empowerment outcomes and political and social changes.
Implementation	Control over decisions essentially rests with outside agent.	Control over decisions is constantly being negotiated.
Terminology	Also known as community-based and social planning programmes.	Also known as community empowerment, community development and community capacity-building programmes.
Evaluation	Evaluation concerned with targets and outcomes often determined by the outside agents.	Evaluation concerned with process and outcomes and inclusion of the participants.

Adapted from Laverack and Labonte, 2000: 256.

and creates what is called a 'bottom-up versus top-down tension' as communities struggle to get their concerns, largely based on gaining more control, heard within traditional programme design.

■ Empowerment and public health programming

A major challenge to the Practitioner is therefore how to accommodate community empowerment (bottom-up) approaches within top-down programming. To achieve this goal the process of community empowerment can be better viewed as a 'parallel track' running alongside the main 'programme or public health track'. The tensions between the two, rather than being conventionally viewed as a top-down versus bottom-up tension, then occur at each stage of the programme cycle, making their resolution practicable. Parallel-tracking also helps to move our thinking on from a simple bottom-up/top-down dichotomy and to formalise bottom-up objectives within more conventional top-down public health programmes. The programming issue at stake is how the public health track and the empowerment track become linked during the progressive stages of the programme cycle. Through 'parallel-tracking' financial, material, human and other resources can be systematically made available to the community in a more empowering way through the design of the programme. The purpose of the programme itself changes to become a pathway through which community empowerment is intentionally developed rather than being viewed as an unexpected benefit of the design.

At the early stages of the programme cycle, the design stage, there are a number of important considerations to promote empowerment including the timeframe, terminology and problem assessment which I next discuss. Conflict resolution is also an important consideration and is discussed later on in this chapter.

To move from a relatively powerless to a more empowered position involves building capacity and to achieve this it is preferable to have a long programme time frame. Too short a time frame runs the real risk of initiating community-level changes, only to end before such changes have reached some degree of sustainability within the community. The empowerment process should therefore start with realistic community issues which are achievable and that can produce visible successes in the short term to sustain interest and promote the progression onto other initiatives. The first opportunity when the 'top-down' and 'bottom-up' tension can begin to be resolved is at the design phase of the programme. Participatory planning approaches allow community involvement and help to resolve conflicts that may arise later during implementation and management. It is at the design phase that the power relationship is established between the Practitioner or their agency, and the other stakeholders of the programme, in particular, the intended beneficiaries. During the design phase of the programme Practitioners must be prepared to listen to what people want, they may not necessarily like what they hear, but they must be committed to initially moving forward and building upon these issues. The role of the Practitioner is to assist the community to define the key concepts, such as community empowerment, to identify their problems and through their own actions to address how they will resolve these problems.

■ Defining the key concepts

Empowerment is widely viewed in the Western literature as a process of capacity building towards a form of power-over that can lead to some people gaining at the expense of others, a zero-sum situation. But as I explain in Chapter 2, the social and cultural perceptions of power and empowerment can be very different in non-westernised countries. The aim of developing a working definition in a programme context is to use terms that have been identified and defined by the clients themselves. These lay interpretations of power and empowerment can then be

Box 3.1 Developing a Working Definition for Community Empowerment

In Fiji, the use of simple qualitative techniques have been shown to identify the key terms in regard to power and empowerment. Unstructured interviews were first used with participants in the programme to identify the headings for power-over or lewa, power-from-within and power-with or kaukauwa. Then through semi-structured interviews the term 'lewa' was further identified to refer to 'chiefly lewa', the control of the village chief and the power-over bestowed at work or in the home. The term kaukauwa is the closest concept in a Fijian context to empowerment. It refers to community strength and unity which can be developed and assisted by its members and can be used to describe the right a person has to do some-thing. Chiefly lewa is a state, a status that is bestowed by birthright or by others in an accepted way and is interdependent on the strength or kaukauwa of the community. It is in the interests of the person with the chiefly lewa and the community to maintain and increase the kaukauwa. The relationship is reciprocal and in this way, the lewa and kaukauwa play an important role in the unity and strength of the community. The kaukauwa may be a mechanism by which the community manage the authority delegated to them by the person with the lewa. It may also be a mechanism used when the community decides to resist and challenge this authority. Although the two terms provide a common understanding this can depend on how they are used. For example, the term kaukauwa in the form 'veivakakaukauwataki' suggests action and a process rather than just a concept and would be a more useful term to use in a programme (Laverack, 1998).

used alongside technical language and terminology so that everyone has a mutual understanding of the programme in which they are involved and towards which they are expected to contribute. The identification of working definitions can be best developed at the beginning of the programme during the design phase. Box 3.1 provides an example of the procedure used to develop a working definition of empowerment in a Fijian context through the use of simple social inquiry techniques to collect and analyse qualitative information. This important professional competence is also discussed in Chapter 7 for the measurement of empowerment.

■ Problem assessment

Problem assessment is a crucial stage in the design of a public health programme that is committed to addressing community issues. The problem assessment approach involves problem mapping or identification, ranking and prioritisation, analysing the causes and solutions and developing a strategic plan to address and resolve them. Too rigid an approach and the programme runs the real risk of becoming top-down and controlling. Too flexible an approach and the programme runs the real risk of becoming delayed or not having a focus and a direction with which to move forward.

Susan Rifkin and Pat Pridmore (2001), two academic commentators on participatory approaches, provide a summary of several different techniques for mapping individual and community problems for increased participation. Mapping is a visual means of providing information in regard to a community problem. The visual aspect helps people to understand the issues at all levels and to find ways in which to solve them. Maps are commonly geographical, concerning the physical layout of a community, or social, identifying the people and where they are situated. Mapping can be done in a collective or on an individual basis (Rifkin and Pridmore, 2001). The purpose is to allow people to better understand, through a textual or a visual means, how they can build their power base (material and social) from an existing position of strength. The role of the Practitioner is to act

---

Box 3.2   Problem Identification through Community Stories

Community stories are a practical exercise to help groups to identify important problems in their community, to help build mutual understanding and power-from-within. The exercise takes between 1 and 2 hours and uses a simple tool called 'unserialised posters' which are prepared in advance of the exercise and are pictures, for example, cuttings from magazines or hand-drawn diagrams. The pictures show a variety of situations relevant to the community such as the building of a new road, a community meeting or a road traffic accident. The group members are asked to select four of the unserialised posters and to develop a story about their community using the pictures. The group is asked to give names to the people and places in the pictures and to give the story a beginning, a middle and an end. The group is then asked to present the story. Other participants are encouraged to ask questions about the story and in particular, the facilitator (the Practitioner) should ask: Are these stories about events in your community? What issues have been raised that could be considered to be problems in your community? How could these problems be solved? What other problems does your community face? The Practitioner keeps a record of the problems that have been identified during the presentation of the story. These points are then used to generate a discussion with the group on what it has learned during the exercise, what were its main problems and what problems it feels could be addressed by the community. The Practitioner can help the community to address its problems by, for example, developing a strategy to address its concerns and by linking the group to organisations or other groups that share the same concerns (Adapted from Wood et al., 1998, p. 24).

as a guide to encourage the community to think critically about what are their own strengths, their access to external resources and their ability to make decisions. In Box 3.2 I provide a practical visual technique, community stories, that can be used to help people in mapping and assessing their own problems.

But not all Practitioners have the skills to use participatory approaches to help others to carry out a problem assessment as described in Box 3.2 and so in Box 3.3 I provide an example of how some Practitioners have used a semi-participatory approach in a school community to help students to identify their problems.

Once the problems have been identified it is the role of the Practitioner to help the community to develop a strategy to rank them and then to move toward decision making and action. Ranking is a simple exercise to 'unpack' the many complex issues that influence peoples lives into its different elements so that they can be placed into a specific order, further analysed and then addressed in a realistic way. Ranking is a way of asking people to prioritise or categorise problems that are important to them. When working with clients who are non-literate, pictures

---

Box 3.3   Problem Identification in a School Community in Scotland

Hillhead primary school is in an inner city area in Glasgow, Scotland with 500 children up to the age of 12 years. The Parents and Teachers Association and children had raised the problem of accidents both inside and outside the school environment. The Practitioners wanted to find out from the children about their perspectives of school safety and how they would like to make it a safer environment as part of the design of a public health intervention.

The younger children were encouraged to describe the safe and unsafe areas of the school and on their journey to and from the school by using a drawing. The older children were shown epidemiological data in a visual format using bar charts, pie charts and graphs of school and road accidents in the Glasgow area. These children were asked what they thought this information meant, why did more accidents happen to boys, why they happened at certain times of the day and in certain places? The children provided very thoughtful answers even raising the issue of reporting bias and this provided a different perspective to the Practitioners. The children were asked for their ideas on how to redesign the school playground and on any new rules that they would like to introduce to help make their school a safer place. The childrens' suggestions included painting the edges of stairs, removing spikes from railings, putting benches in playgrounds where children could rest as a quiet area away from the rough and tumble of the playground and staggering playtimes to allow the younger children to play and to avoid older children. The Practitioner could then use the ideas put forward by the participants as a part of a planning process for community actions, supported by an outside agency (Roberts, 1998).

Box 3.4 Analysing Community Problems: The Story with a Gap

The 'story with a gap' is used to stimulate discussion about the causes of and the solutions to priority health problems that the community has already identified.

Each group is given two large pictures. One picture shows the before situation of a community priority problem, for example, a road traffic accident. The group is asked to develop a story about their community and the problems that they have encountered due to traffic in their area. The participants are encouraged to make the story realistic by including the names of places and people.

The second picture shows the after situation, for example, slow moving traffic regulated by traffic lights or speed bumps. The group is asked to develop a story which explains how this improvement has occurred. The stories that they develop will 'fill the gap' between the two pictures. The group members are asked to recount their story and the content is discussed to identify possible pathways to the solutions.

This exercise allows participants to generate ideas about how the community can organise itself to find solutions to problems which they feel have a high priority. The Practitioner facilitators this process of discovery and is part of building specific skills necessary for community capacity (Srinivasan, 1993).

or drawings can be used instead of words to develop a ranked list. The prioritised list can then be scored, giving the highest score to the issue at the top of the list and the lowest score to the issue at the bottom of the list. The Practitioner discusses the reasons why one issue is scored higher than another in the list. The next step is for the Practitioner to help the community to begin to analyse the prioritised list. In Box 3.4 I provide the example of 'story with a gap', a simple visual technique to enable people to analyse important problems shared by their community and then to develop strategies to address them.

I next provide an example of empowerment in maternal and new born health to illustrate how 'parallel-tracking' (WHO, 2007) can be used in public health programming (see Figure 3.1) to accommodate both top-down and bottom-up approaches.

■ 'Parallel-tracking' empowerment into maternal and newborn health

☐ Setting programme objectives

Objective setting within conventional top-down programming is usually centred around disease prevention, a reduction in morbidity and mortality and lifestyle

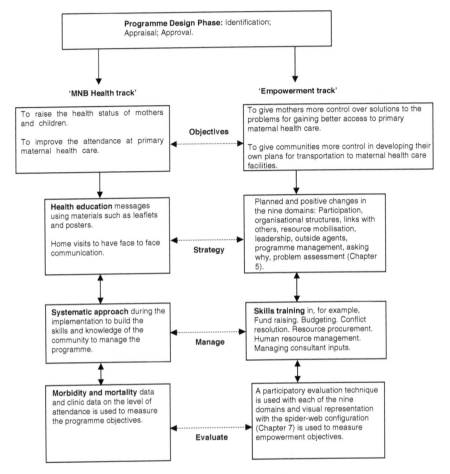

Figure 3.1 Parallel-tracking maternal and newborn health programmes Adapted from WHO, 2007.

management such as a change in specific health related behaviours. The issue is how to give empowerment objectives an equal priority with the disease prevention objectives and to reflect this in the parallel-track.

The Practitioner must firstly ascertain from the participants what are their problems, discussed earlier, and this information is then used to set the empowerment objectives. Empowerment objectives need to be flexible as they are likely to change as the experiences of the programme participants also change over time. However, they also need to be achievable and measurable and this can be facilitated by the Practitioner to assist the community to narrow its focus towards more immediate and resolvable issues. For example, in maternal and new born health the two sets of objectives might include:

- **Programme objectives**
  - To raise the health status of mothers and children.
  - To improve the attendance at primary maternal health care.

- **Empowerment objectives**
  - To give mothers more control-over solutions to the problems for gaining better access to primary maternal health care.
  - To give communities more control in developing their own plans for trans portation to maternal health care facilities.

☐ Developing the strategic approach

It is important that the strategic approach used by the programme is paralleled by strategies that build community empowerment. In this example the objectives are to raise the health status of mothers and children and to improve the attendance of mothers at primary maternal health care facilities. To achieve the objectives the programme might typically employ communication and behaviour change strategies, for example, health education materials, talks by nurses to mothers, visits to households by Practitioners to discuss the importance of attending primary maternal health facilities.

Strategies for strengthening the empowerment of mothers to gain more control in regard to primary maternal health care might include building the capacity of women's groups to address, for example, better transportation services or collective fund raising to support the cost of child birth and care. The role of the Practitioner is to support the process of capacity building partly by attending to the dynamics that underpin the different points along the empowerment continuum discussed in Chapter 5. And partly by strengthening competencies in each of the nine empowerment 'domains', discussed in Chapter 6.

It is important to set short-term performance goals, for example, the development of local leadership skills or the formation of a women's group, because these achievable successes can help to motivate people toward the longer-term maternal health objectives. The progress should be periodically reviewed with the participants to reflect on their success and failures.

☐ Programme management and implementation

The programme management process is traditionally concerned with planning, organising, leading and controlling the utilisation of resources, both human and material, to achieve its objectives (O'Connor and Parker, 1995). The person who controls, or has power-over, this process determines the direction and sometimes the success of achieving the objectives. In more general terms management is concerned with effectiveness, the extent to which objectives are achieved, and efficiency, the way in which the objectives are achieved compared to other means (Ewles and Simnett, 2003).

The role of the Practitioner is to be sympathetic to community ownership and involvement to help make the management process an empowering experience for the participants. This can be achieved by encouraging participants to play an increasing role in programme management, for example, activities such as reporting, budgeting and the procurement of resources. In order to have the confidence to undertake these responsibilities the participants may have to acquire specific skills through training in, for example, proposal writing, creative problem solving and conducting effective group meetings. Table 3.2 provides a list of relevant skills training for community members that can be systematically incorporated by the Practitioner as part of the management plan during the timeframe of the programme.

☐   Evaluation of the programme

The final stage in the programme cycle is normally an evaluation of the outcomes often set against the objectives, although mid-term evaluations and monitoring can also be carried out. In 'parallel-tracking' the aim is that both the programme

Table 3.2   Developing skills in public health programme planning and management

Programme phase	Skills training
Design	• Analysis of epidemiological data. • Identification of community problems. • Appraisal of programme design.
Objective Setting	• Writing SMART objectives. • Logframe development.
Strategic Approach	• Strategies to empower individuals, groups and communities. • Public health models and theories. • Interpersonal communication. • Workshop facilitation. • Conducting effective group meetings and public presentation.
Programme management	• Fund raising. • Budgeting. • Conflict resolution. • Resource procurement. • Human resource management.
Evaluation	• Participatory Rural Appraisal techniques. • Qualitative research methods. • Quantitative research methods.

Adapted from Laverack, 2007, p. 57.

and empowerment objectives are evaluated. Empowerment, as an outcome, may not occur until after the time frame of a top-down programme, normally two to five years, has been completed. Thus, the evaluation of community empowerment within a programme context can more appropriately assessed as a process as well as specific outcomes. Programme success in terms of empowerment is best judged in terms of how the participants, through a self-assessment, experienced improvements in their lives and health. The evaluation therefore needs to employ participatory methods that draw upon the experiences and knowledge of the programme participants. There is also the need to be systematic in the way in which we evaluate community empowerment, how we compare the information collected overtime, between respondents and between communities within the same programme and how we present and interpret this information. In Chapter 7 I describe the systematic evaluation of community empowerment and discuss how the evaluation can be visually represented using the spider-web configuration and how this information can be used to quickly interpret the strengths and weaknesses of a community.

■ Resolving conflict

Conflict can be a negative ingredient of the empowerment process by taking attention away from important issues, by dividing community groups and by undermining individuals' power-from-within. However if managed correctly it can also be a positive ingredient. Dealing with conflict in a positive way can resolve disputes, help to release emotions and anxieties and make the community address sensitive issues whilst at the same time improving co-operation and communication. The beginnings of conflict are often caused by poor communication between individual stakeholders and between interest groups, weak local leadership, internal struggles to gain access to limited resources, struggles between the powerless and those seen to hold the power and the uncertainty of Practitioners about their role in resolving conflict (Laverack, 2005).

In Box 3.5 I provide an exercise that can help both Practitioners and clients to understand the strategies and tactics that can be used to help reflect on their own reactions in a position of power imbalance. In this exercise the power is represented by the allocation of resources. Whilst the difference in allocation is minor this is representative of more meaningful ones that can result in the participants making connections to other areas in their lives where they may be unaware of the disparities of access to power (Coleman, 2000). The exercise can be used as part of a training activity for Practitioners or as a means of demonstrating to their clients the disruptive effect that conflict can have on a community.

In conflict situations, those with the power-over tend to try to dominate, to use pressure tactics and to offer few concessions and this can make it difficult to reach a negotiated agreement that is satisfactory to all parties. Those who are in a powerless position become alienated and are presented with two main options for them to gain power: (1) to resist by increasing their own resources, organisation and mobilisation and using this in tactics of disobedience and activism; (2) to induce

Box 3.5 Positions of Power and Conflict

The trainer organises the tables in the room into two areas each to accommodate half of the participants. In one area, the table is provided with markers, coloured pens, paints, coloured paper, scissors, magazines and other decorative items. In the other area, the table is provided with one sheet of blank paper and two lead pencils. The participants are invited back into the room and randomly allocated to one of the two areas.

The two groups are given the same objective: to develop a working definition of power and empowerment. They are informed that once the groups have finished the exercise they will be asked to display their definitions and a vote will be taken by everyone in the room to select the best and most attractive definition. The groups are then asked to begin the exercise and the trainers actively support the group with most resources whilst actively ignoring the group with the least resources.

The definitions are displayed and a discussion held to discuss the best definition including the use of colour, attractiveness and technical content. The participants are also asked to discuss the dynamics of the two groups, their feelings and how they interacted during the exercise. Participants may be unaware of the disparities in resource allocation, may have tried to persuade the other group to give them extra resources or even to take resources without asking. These points are discussed in relation to the issue of power and conflict.

Adapted from Coleman, 2000, pp. 127–8.

those with power to use it more benevolently and to be sympathetic to the helplessness and position of inequality of those with less power (Coleman, 2000). To enable their clients to gain more power-over in (1) above or to be in a better position of power to negotiate in (2) above requires a strategic approach by Practitioners in a programme context to resolve conflict. These strategies include: Providing training for conflict management; Developing communication tools to better disseminate information (discussed in Chapter 4); Using listening to clarify understanding (Chapter 4); Eliminating power-over to build power-with others (Chapter 2); Providing a facilitated dialogue to resolve issues (Chapter 7); Ranking the issues needed to map concerns and positions of power (Chapters 3 and 4); Naming personal issues that cloud the picture and assess the problem in its broader context by using approaches of critical awareness and thinking (Chapter 4).

Practitioners cannot be expected to use all these strategies in their everyday work but they can choose to adopt some in a situation of conflict when this is creating a barrier to moving forward. The Practitioner can play an important role in resolving conflict by simply assessing the situation, being a good listener and inviting stakeholder participation to clarify areas of conflict. An example of resolving cross-cultural differences is provided in Box 3.6 in the 'Resolving Differences – Building Communities Project' in the UK.

Box 3.6 'Resolving Differences – Building Communities Project' in the UK

The 'Resolving Differences – Building Communities Project' started after conflict erupted in 2001 between groups of Somalian and African-Carribbean youth in Leicester, UK. The Somalians were settled as new immigrants into poor socio-economic areas occupied by the African-Caribbean community and this created inter-ethnic tensions. The Somalians found it difficult to assimilate into the British culture, had language constraints and could not easily access available services. The Project established a steering group made up of stakeholders from the two communities with the task of coordinating the management and implementation. The main purpose of the Project was to clarify the views and opinions of the two groups about one another through workshops and focus group discussions. Local people were trained and employed as cross-cultural facilitators to provide peer education, mediation and recruit some 400 young volunteers. In particular, it was the role of the facilitators, assisted by Practitioners, that led to a reduction in prejudice and who managed to directly avoid conflict over the following months because of their interaction and attempts to build cohesion (renewal.net, 2008).

The 'Aik Saath Project' is a similar project which was started to address inter-ethnic tension and outbreaks of conflict between the Sikh and Muslim youth in Slough, UK. Again the role of locally recruited and trained facilitators in conflict resolution played a major role in reducing tensions, such as the number of playground fights between Sikhs and Muslims, and in building a working relationship with street gangs. The Project also used local conflict resolution groups and worked in schools to identify and address the key issues causing the tensions. The conflict resolution groups were made up of students from each year and provided an important entry point into the school and into the issues facing youth on inter-ethnic conflict. The groups provided a bridge between the Practitioners and their clients, the youth, and so it was important to carefully manage their development. The Project found that in order to develop a conflict resolution group it was necessary to: carefully select the targeted youth; work with existing community-based organisations in contact with the youth; invest in young people to act as facilitators and provide them with outreach resources; have mechanisms to value their input; engage with key public sector agencies; and have a realistic timeframe to achieve your aims (Renewal.net, 2008).

Conflict resolution does not have to be a specialist area of work especially when the issue of disagreement is not complicated and can be resolved by a simple clarification and discussion of the main concerns. This is a process that can be facilitated by the Practitioner using participatory approaches to promote discussion. In Box 3.7 I provide the example of a simple exercise that can be used by Practitioners to help resolve conflict by, first, mapping the main questions and

Box 3.7 Defining the Issues of Conflict

To carry out this exercise the Practitioner should have some prior idea about the key questions that will be asked and some of the solutions that can be discussed. This will help the Practitioner to focus the discussion on the practical and not on the personal points. The Practitioner should be able to firstly define the issues and the problem areas of the conflict in neutral terms that all participants can agree upon.

1. The participants are asked to construct a list of key questions about the conflict, the potential solutions to the questions.
2. The participants and the Practitioner next identify sources of the information regarding each of the key questions, for example, web sites, local leaders, government officials, that are necessary to move into a problem-solving stage.
3. The participants are asked to prepare a summary of the conflict by comparing each question with a possible solution and a source of information. This can be usefully summarised in a table in a compact format.
4. After a period of discussion between the different parties the table can be rewritten to highlight how major changes in one conflict alters over time as circumstances change.

It is necessary to note that this type of a problem-solving exercise is not a negotiation or a political commitment, it is merely a commitment to further analysis and discussion.
Adapted from Mitchell and Banks, 1998, p. 31.

issues held between the different stakeholders involved and then by developing strategies to address each concern.

Next Chapter 4 addresses how Practitioners can work specifically with individuals to help them to gain power, and in particular, enabling Practitioners to become better communicators, increasing the critical awareness of their clients and by fostering an empowering working relationship.

Chapter 4

Helping individuals to gain power

■ Overcoming powerlessness

Helping individual clients to gain power begins by building their power-from-within and helping them to participate in 'interest' groups and community organisations. It is collective, rather than individual, empowerment that eventually brings about the broader social and political changes that are necessary to address inequalities in health. Individuals achieve these goals through their involvement in social networks, by mobilising resources and by improving their personal and collective competencies.

As discussed in Chapter 2, powerlessness is the absence of power, whether imagined or real, and is an individual concept with the expectancy that the behaviour of a person (or group) cannot determine the outcomes they seek (Kieffer, 1984). Powerlessness is a barrier to gaining power and something that both Practitioners and their clients can experience. For Practitioners this might mean the actions of an authoritative doctor controlling the decisions made by a nurse in an outpatient clinic or a senior nurse micro-managing the work of the ward nurses in a hospital. For a client this might mean being shown indifference from a Practitioner about their needs or being excluded in collaborating about their care planning. It is important that the Practitioner is first able to recognise his/her own position of powerlessness. As I discuss in Chapter 2, before Practitioners can empower others they must first empower themselves by understanding the sources of their own power.

The exercise in Box 4.1 allows Practitioners to begin to think critically, discuss and support one another in regard to their own positions of powerlessness in a work setting. The exercise can be carried out in small groups or on an individual basis.

It is important that the Practitioner is able to identify their own power base and then to develop a strategy to address the situation before moving forward to help their clients to overcome their powerlessness. In Box 4.2 I provide an exercise on weaning practices to help Practitioners to understand how they can use their power base to help, in this example, a young mother. In many countries women do not make decisions in isolation from the context of their lives and this often involves asking other family members for advice. In this example, Heidi, a young mother, has been advised by a nurse Practitioner to exclusively breastfeed her child until it is six months old. The nurse Practitioner has explained the nutritional, protective and child spacing benefits of breastfeeding as well as showing her how to initiate skin contact and hold the child to encourage her to feed and bond with the mother. However, Heidi's mother is encouraging her to wean the baby at three months by feeding it porridge. This is Heidi's first child and she is very anxious about giving her baby the best start in life but feels under considerable family pressure to feed the child porridge. Her sense of powerless has made Heidi feel depressed and anxious about the safety of her child. Heidi feels powerless about this situation and asks another nurse Practitioner to help with this decision-making process.

Box 4.1 Examining Positions of Professional Powerlessness

The Practitioners are asked to produce a description (written or pictorial) of themselves in a position where the Director of Nursing (or another person in authority to themselves) has power-over them in their work setting.

The Practitioners are then asked:
How do you feel in this situation?
What is the basis for your sense of powerlessness?
How can they change the situation to make themselves feel more comfortable?
What simple strategies could they apply to empower themselves?

The Practitioners are encouraged to discuss their answers with the whole group and for the facilitator to develop a discussion around some of the key issues raised. The facilitator can write the main points and strategies onto a board so that all the Practitioners can see the outcome of the discussion.

Box 4.2 Powerlessness and Weaning Practices

What should the nurse Practitioner do to help empower Heidi?

After discussing the example of Heidi in groups the participants are asked to share their ideas on how to help Heidi based on the introduction to the concepts of power and empowerment. These ideas can be written on a white-board or large sheet of paper to display them to other participants.

Possible discussion points:

1. The nurse Practitioner uses her authority and professional status to lend credibility to Heidi's concerns.
2. Mentoring the woman to identify her own power-bases (social support, family, friends) to strengthen her power-from-within.
3. Using her power-over (status, authority) the nurse Practitioner can advocate to the head of the family ('I'll do this, but only if you'll consider how to learn to do it yourselves...') the nurse Practitioner exercises her control with the intent of increasing the power-from-within of Heidi and her family.

Individual clients need to have the self-confidence to participate and interact in a group setting in such a way as to make their opinions and concerns count. As discussed in Chapter 2, self-confidence and self-esteem are characteristics of power-from-within. To build power-from-within, the Practitioners use strategies to increase feelings of value and a sense of control in their clients. Whilst the ability of the Practitioner to be an effective communicator can be closely linked to the way in which people feel about themselves, individuals become more powerful through their own sense of worth rather than from a simple transfer of information.

There are many strategies that can help individuals to gain power and to build their power-from-within and whilst it would be unrealistic for Practitioners to attempt to use them all, here I select key approaches under the following three headings that can be used as part of their everyday work:

1. Practitioners as more effective communicators;
2. Increasing the critical awareness of individual clients; and
3. Fostering an empowering professional-client relationship.

■ Practitioners as more effective communicators

Practitioners often use health education, health communication and Information, Education and Communication (IEC) strategies in their everyday work to impart information to their clients. Practitioners also use communication to advocate on behalf of their clients or to mediate between conflicting interest groups. Health education is aimed at informing people to influence their individual decision making centred on lifestyle choices, whereas health promotion aims at complementary social and political actions that facilitate broader changes in peoples' lives to enhance health (Green and Kreuter, 1991). In practice, health promotion encompasses health education and health communication approaches and can be viewed as an umbrella term for a range of educational and health promoting activities (Ewles and Simnett, 2003). For example, health education around tobacco issues might include school-based awareness programmes or smoking cessation courses. Health promotion around tobacco issues extends to legislation restricting access to tobacco products, bans on advertising and retail displays and legislation restricting where smoking might be allowed. Health communication is the exchange of information in regard to health issues to raise awareness, develop a dialogue and to educate people. The main purpose of health communication is to influence health-related behaviours. Likewise, IEC is a general term for communication activities to promote a variety of issues including health. What all these approaches have in common is that they are based on the need to make Practitioners more effective communicators.

The communication can be individually focused on a one (the Practitioner)-to-one (the client) basis, for example, a doctor talking to a patient in his/her surgery. The communication can also be focused to reach a larger audience, for example, a group discussion that is used to develop a dialogue between a nurse and a group of mothers waiting at a well baby clinic. Communication can help individuals to gain more control over their lives by providing:

- an increase in health knowledge and skills, for example, for the preparation of an oral rehydration solution;
- information that is necessary for them to make a specific 'informed choice or decision' to have greater control in regard to health, for example, the benefits of breast feeding or immunisation;
- an increase in the understanding of the underlying causes of their lack of power, for example, unemployment and a low income.

■ One-to-one communication

One-to-one communication is important because this allows a dialogue to develop between the client and the Practitioner. The dialogue is often based on a sharing of knowledge and experiences in a two-way communication that is necessary to help individuals to better retain information, to clarify personal issues and to develop skills. Verbal communication is probably the most common channel of relaying information between the Practitioner and the client and can be either one-way (Practitioner to client) or two-way (sharing information between Practitioner and client). Situations where one-to-one communication takes place include providing physiotherapy advice to an individual and counseling someone on a sensitive issue such as the result of a medical test.

The relationship of Practitioners with their clients can be influenced by the level of control (power) that they have through their choice of communication style. It is important to emphasise that the choice of the communication style is usually at the discretion of the Practitioner, who decides, based on the circumstances and the type of client, what is most ethically acceptable. For example, using a controlling approach such as a direct instruction to make the client take a prescribed medication might be seen as an unethical imposition of the Practitioner's values. This can be reinforced through non-verbal communication, for example, body language, posture and facial expressions. Whenever possible the Practitioner should consider a communication style that is non-controlling such as the GATHER approach outlined in Box 4.3 or follow a simple procedure of listening, giving advice and obtaining and providing feedback.

■ Learning to listen

Listening is an active process and the Practitioner needs to focus on what the individual is saying and if necessary to help the speaker to express his/her feelings or to give an opinion on an issue. The following is a simple exercise that allows Practitioners to think carefully about how they communicate with their clients and is designed to illustrate better communication between the Practitioner and a

Box 4.3 The GATHER Approach to One-to-One Communication

G Greet the clients make them feel comfortable, show respect, trust and empathy.

A Ask them about their problem: Help them to talk about their problems and needs, listen to them and encourage their feedback.

T Tell them any relevant information: Provide technical information about their health issue, use simple language and focus on the important points.

H Help them to make decisions: By exploring the options to their particular circumstances and by developing a realistic action plan.

E Explain any misunderstandings: Ask questions and clarify any issues raised.

R Return to follow up on them: Revisit, make a reappointment or refer the clients to another practitioner to ensure that the issues were understood and acted upon. Obtain and give feedback.

Adapted from Hubley, 1993, p. 97.

woman in regard to preparation for a home delivery (WHO, 2007). The participants are divided into groups of three people. The group is asked to designate someone who will be the 'Practitioner', someone who will be the 'mother' and someone who will be an impartial 'observer'. The role of the 'observer' is to watch the interaction between the 'Practitioner' and the 'mother' without making any comments or interruptions to their conversation. The 'observer' uses Exercise Sheet 1 (Table 4.1) to record the level of interaction and communication between the 'Practitioner' and the 'mother'. The 'Practitioner' and the 'mother' are given Exercise Sheet 2 (Table 4.2) and asked to carefully consider the circumstances. They are not told how to do this. The mode of interaction is decided upon by the two people and this automatically sets up a power dynamic between the 'Practitioner' and the 'mother'. This dynamic will vary depending on the power-from-within and power-over of the two people. After the exercise has finished the participants discuss their experiences as the 'Practitioner', the 'mother' and the 'observer' in one group.

The facilitator can ask, for example:

1. What did they feel about the level of one to one communication?
2. Did the 'Practitioner' use empowering language?
3. Did the 'Practitioner' listen to the 'mother'?
4. Did the 'Practitioner' facilitate the 'mother' to help her to make her own decisions?

Exercise Sheet 3 (Table 4.3) provides an example of some potential actions that can be developed by mothers to plan for a delivery and is shared with participants after the exercise. The Practitioner and mother are to sit together to complete the

Table 4.1   Exercise Sheet 1. The communication skills checklist

Did the 'Practitioner?	Yes	No	Comments from observer
Introduce themselves to the mother.			
Use the mother's name.			
Greet the mother.			
Explain their role and purpose.			
Ensure that the mother was comfortable.			
Establish and maintain eye contact.			
Listen to what the mother was saying.			
Use open-ended questions.			
Inform the mother that information would be recorded.			
Maintain interest in what the mother was saying during note taking.			
Identify and respond to verbal and non-verbal cues.			
Give appropriate and accurate advice.			
Provide a summary of what was said and agreed.			
Obtain feedback from the mother.			
Give a pleasant thank you and farewell.			

Adapted from Lloyd and Bor, 2004: 190.

actions identified to resolve the concern and place them in order of priority. The first suggested action has been provided in Table 4.2 to encourage discussion.

When giving advice the Practitioner is exerting his/her expert and legitimate power to persuade the client into actually accepting a subservient role relationship. The relationship grants the Practitioner the right to prescribe advice while

Table 4.2   Exercise Sheet 2. Learning to listen

Column 1. Priority concern expressed by the mother.	Column 2. Actions identified to resolve this concern.
Do not have a plan for the birth of their child? (Where will the birth take place? By whom? How will you get there?)	Develop a birth plan with clear roles and responsibilities and shared decision making for a husband, wife and family.

Table 4.3 Exercise Sheet 3. Learning to listen

Column 1. Priority concern expressed by the mother.	Column 2 Actions identified to resolve this concern.
Do not have a plan for the birth of their child? (Where will the birth take place? By whom? How will you get there?)	Develop a birth plan with clear roles and responsibilities and shared decision making for man, wife and family.
	Identify who will take the mother to the place of delivery and who will stay with her during labour.
	Access to information about what will happen during labour, the danger signs leading up to giving birth and postnatal self-care.
	Have adequate supplies for the birth (new blade in clean cover, clean thread, at least five cloths, washed and dried in the sun, change of clothes, food and drink).

Adapted from WHO, 2007.

the client accepts an obligation to comply with the advice. This can relate to a range of different types of information and behaviour change for a healthier lifestyle and the Practitioner may also have to use their power-over in a form of dominance to control people's choices. This is sometimes a necessary communication style when, for example, giving a precise instruction such as the self-treatment of a wound by the patient to ensure their compliance.

Obtaining and giving feedback enables the Practitioner to clarify what the client wants, that they have understood previous communication or retained skills. This may mean obtaining feedback based on specific information using closed questions that require short factual (yes/no) answers or based on an open form of questioning to provide fuller answers.

Giving feedback is important for the achievement of effective communication and in particular positive feedback that reinforces the strengths of the client's knowledge or skills level. The client is encouraged to share his/her concerns, feelings and opinions but the discussion is directed by the Practitioner. To facilitate this process the Practitioner can use 'people centred' approaches such as the patient-centred clinical method discussed in Chapter 2.

An assessment of the procedure of communication involving listening, giving advice and obtaining and providing feedback can be an important part of the learning process for the Practitioner. The communication skills checklist provided in Table 4.1 can be used by trainers in role-play or practice sessions. The Practitioner is observed by the trainer, or by another Practitioner, who completes each section of the checklist and then provides feedback. The identified strengths of inter-personal communication and the areas that need further work are then discussed to improve the ability of the Practitioner.

■ Combining communication channels

Communication strategies can be made to be more effective for increasing knowledge by using a combination of channels as a part of the same intervention. The most commonly used channels are the mass media, print materials, one-to-one communication, popular media and school-based activities. The mass media includes radio, television, audio-cassettes and telecommunications such as the internet. These approaches are used to reach a large audience rapidly and at a relatively low cost. Print materials include posters, leaflets, booklets and flip charts and these can be used as a part of one-to-one communication to assist the transfer of information and skills when working with both literate and non-literate populations. The picture material is used to generate a two-way discussion between the Practitioner and the clients and is especially useful in a teaching environment such as with a group of school children. School-based activities include participatory exercises for life skills, competitions and contests and counseling (one-to-one communication) covering a range of issues.

Communication strategies used in public health programmes have traditionally been implemented as interventions relying on only one or two channels, for example, a mass media campaign on road safety. This is because the frequency and design of communication activities has been largely determined by the availability of resources. Figure 4.1 offers a simple approach to combine different communication channels as a part of the same intervention. The communication intervention is represented as a triangle. Each point of the triangle represents a different communication channel that is implemented on a regular basis as part of the intervention, for example, weekly radio broadcasts, the distribution of leaflets and counseling sessions between the Practitioner and a client. The centre of the triangle represents an 'opportunistic channel', such as community theatre, one that is used when the opportunity arises, usually when people congregate in a public place, for example, at clinics, in shopping malls or leisure centres. The combination of channels can be changed, to develop different communication interventions, and are designed to be used together to strengthen the approach. For example, formal didactic methods can be made more participatory and more empowering when used with teaching aids such as picture cards and flipcharts. It is important that the target audience(s) is clearly identified and that the message content is specific to each target audience. The message content must be reinforced by being consistently delivered to the target audiences through different channels of communication. The materials must be attractive in design, well presented clear and entertaining to appeal to the target audiences. The approach should be low cost so that production and distribution can be reasonably sustained, for example, by using low cost leaflets for clients to take home and read.

Figure 4.1   Combining communication channels

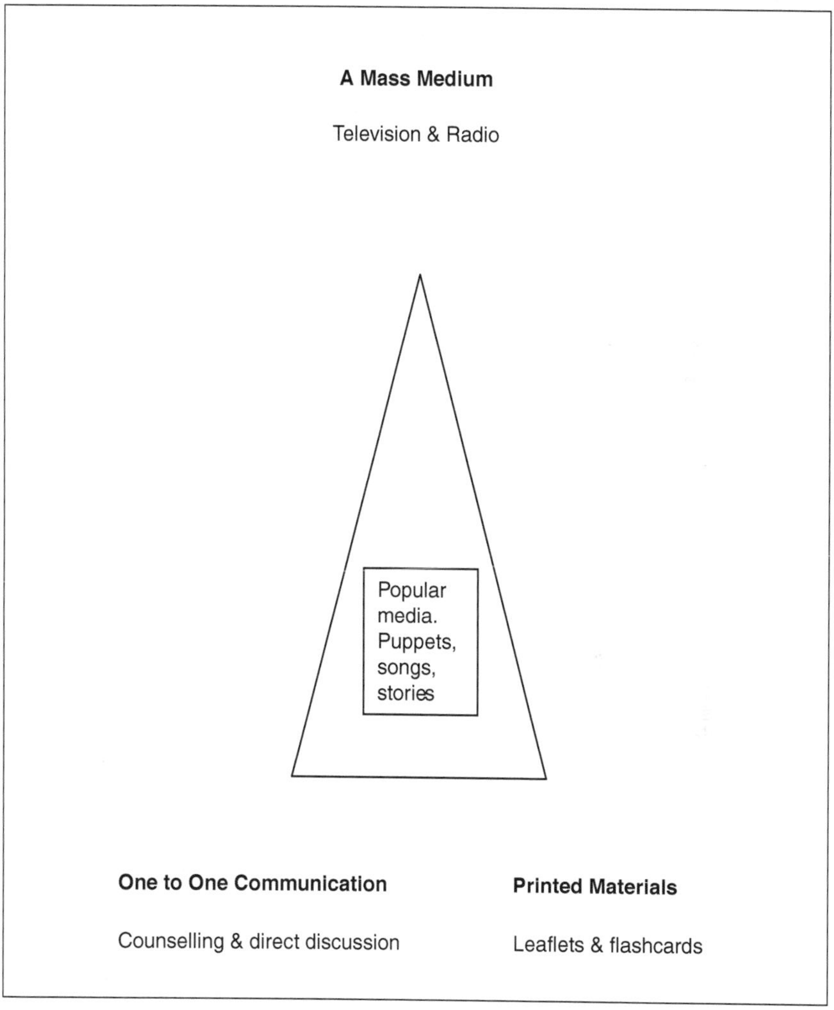

A Mass Medium

Television & Radio

Popular
media.
Puppets,
songs,
stories

One to One Communication   Printed Materials

Counselling & direct discussion   Leaflets & flashcards

Adapted from Laverack and Dap, 2004, p. 367.

■ Increasing the critical awareness of individual clients

Helping individuals to gain power ultimately involves their ability to make and
carry out choices. This often begins by increasing their critical awareness. I define

critical awareness here as 'the ability of the individual to reflect on the assumptions underlying his/her state of health and on actions to achieve alternative behaviours, actions or styles of living'. Critical awareness is a process of learning through discussion, reflection and action. Here I describe three practical exercises that Practitioners can use in their everyday work to strengthen critical awareness: strategies for decision making; Photovoice and health literacy.

■ Strategies for decision making

Choice, or the ability to exercise control over decisions, is the simplest form of power. Strategies for better decision making about, for example, different health options can be a very empowering tool for Practitioners to use when working with individuals. Decision making is a highly complex procedure and a practical approach to promote the basic principles of this process is outlined below. This approach was developed (Laverack, 2003) to promote decision-making skills with individuals and groups and has been field tested in a number of different cultural contexts. Here I use the example of helping an individual client to develop decision-making skills that will give them more control over their desire to improve their health by stopping smoking in the next six months.

☐   Step 1   Ranking key options

Individuals first make a list or ranking of the key options covering their particular health concern. The Practitioner can help by providing specific and accurate technical information to answer any questions about the issue. Susan Rifkin and Pat Pridmore (2001) discuss several techniques to help Practitioners to identify the concerns of their individual clients including preference ranking; pair-wise ranking; matrix scoring; and well-being or wealth ranking. Each can be used in a participatory manner to suit different client needs or used together to provide cross-checking information. The ranking must come from the individuals without them being led or coerced by the Practitioner. If the number of ranked options is large, the Practitioner can assist the individuals to produce a prioritised list, for example, a ranked list for an individual's health options might include:

1. To stop smoking in the next six months;
2. To do more exercise;
3. To lose weight;
4. To eat more healthily.

A ranking of the different choices as set out in Step 1 is in itself insufficient to empower individuals who must also have the ability to transform this information into decisions and actions. This is achieved through developing a decision-making matrix for positive changes in each of the prioritised areas using:

Step 2   Decisions on the key actions to be taken;
Step 3   Decisions on the key activities for each action taken and;
Step 4   The identification of resources.

☐   Step 2   Decisions on the key actions to be taken

The individual is asked to decide on how the situation can be improved for each prioritised area. The purpose is to firstly identify the most feasible actions that will improve the present situation and then to provide a lead into a more detailed strategy in Step 3 outlining the activities. This information is placed in column 2 of the matrix in Table 4.4.

Taking the first ranked health option in Step 1 (To stop smoking in the next six months) the decisions on the key actions to be taken might include:

- Remove all cigarettes from the home and workplace;
- To attend motivation classes to help to stop smoking;
- To use a substitute for smoking such as chewing gum or nicotine patches.

☐   Step 3   Decisions on the key activities for each action taken

The person is next asked to consider in practice the most feasible actions that can be carried out and in particular to identify specific activities, to sequence activities in order to make an improvement and to set a realistic time frame including any significant personal benchmarks or targets. These are placed in column 3 of the matrix. Continuing from the example in Step 2 the activities to implement the identified actions to stop smoking might include the following:

- Collect all cigarettes in house and dispose;
- Do not purchase any more cigarettes;
- Identify local classes. Make time to attend one class per week. Identify a friend to attend initial classes for support;
- Discuss best alternative products with a doctor or pharmacist. Make an appointment to speak with a doctor in the next seven days;
- Buy product from pharmacy. Take on a prescribed basis for the next three months.

☐ Step 4   Identification of resources

The person next identifies the resources that are necessary to implement the actions they have identified in column 3. The Practitioner can help the individual to map the necessary resources, for example, information, finance and social support. To undertake the actions to stop smoking might include:

- The availability of local self-motivation class;
- Money to pay for classes and time to attend the classes;
- Access to a pharmacy or Practitioner to discuss the best options for a smoking substitute and;
- Money to purchase substitute products.

☐ The decision-making matrix

The strategy for decision making can be represented by using a simplified matrix based on the logical framework system developed for the purposes of programme design, monitoring and evaluation (Cracknell, 1996). In Table 4.4 the ranking is placed in the left hand side column followed by sequential columns for:

1. Prioritising the key health issues;
2 Decisions on the key actions to be taken;
3. Decisions on the key activities for each action taken and;
4. The identification of resources.

The matrix provides a summary of the decisions and actions to be undertaken by the individual. This can provide the basis for an 'informal contract' between the Practitioner and the individual. It identifies specific tasks or responsibilities usually set against a timeframe based on the period identified as being realistic, for example, to stop smoking this was given as six months. It also identifies the resources or assistance that will be required to fulfil these tasks and responsibilities, within the agreed timeframe, by both the Practitioner and the client.

■ Photovoice

Paulo Freire (1973) originally developed his ideas on building awareness through learning or education in literacy programmes in the 1950s for slum dwellers and peasants in Brazil. The central premise is that education is not neutral but is influenced by the context of one's life. People become the subjects of their own learning involving critical reflection and analysis of their personal circumstances. To achieve this, Freire proposed a group dialogue approach to share ideas and experiences and to promote critical thinking by posing problems to allow people

Table 4.4 The decision-making matrix: stop smoking in the next six months

Step 1. Priority	Step 2. Key decisions	Step 3. Key activities	Step 4. Resources
To stop smoking for smoking in the next six months.	Remove all cigarettes from the home and workplace; To attend motivation classes to help to stop smoking; To use a substitute to smoking such as chewing gum or nicotine patches.	Collect all cigarettes in house and dispose. Do not purchase any more cigarettes; Identify local classes. Make time to attend one class per week. Identify a friend to attend initial classes for support; Discuss best alternative products with a doctor or pharmacist. Make an appointment to speak with a doctor in the next seven days; Buy product from pharmacy. Take on a prescribed basis for the next three months.	The availability of local self-motivation class; Money to pay for classes and time to attend the classes; Access to a pharmacy or Practitioner to discuss the best options for a smoking substitute and; Money to purchase substitute products.

to uncover the root causes of their powerlessness. This is an ongoing interaction between the Practitioner and their client in a cycle of action/reflection/action and often leads to collective social and political activity (Freire, 1973). This approach does involve a considerable commitment from the client to be able to gradually understand the causes of their powerlessness and to develop realistic actions to begin to resolve the situation.

Photovoice is a process by which people can identify, represent, and enhance their community through a specific photographic technique based on the principles of Paulo Freire. It entrusts cameras to the hands of people to enable them to act as recorders, and potential catalysts for social action and change, in their own communities. It uses the immediacy of the visual image and accompanying stories to furnish evidence and to promote an effective, participatory means of sharing expertise to create healthful public policy.

Photovoice has two main goals:

- To enable people to record and reflect their community's strengths and concerns;

- To promote critical dialogue and knowledge about personal and community issues through large and small group discussions of photographs.

People using Photovoice engage in a three-stage process that provides the foundation for analysing the pictures they have taken:

Stage 1 Selecting: Choosing those photographs that most accurately reflect the community's concerns and assets. So that people can lead the discussion, it is they who choose the photographs. They select photographs they considered most significant, or simply like best, from each roll of film they had taken.

Stage 2 Contextualising or story telling: The participatory approach also generates the second stage, contextualising or storytelling. This occurs in the process of group discussion, suggested by the acronym VOICE, voicing our individual and collective experience. Photographs alone, considered outside the context of their own voices and stories, would contradict the essence of photovoice. People describe the meaning of their images in small and large group discussions.

Stage 3 Codifying: The participatory approach gives multiple meanings to singular images and thus frames the third stage, codifying. In this stage, participants may identify three types of dimensions that arise from the dialogue process: issues, themes, or theories. The individual or group may codify issues when the concerns targeted for action are pragmatic, immediate, and tangible. This is the most direct application of the analysis. The individual or group may also codify themes and patterns, or develop theories that are grounded in a more systematic analysis of the images.

Photovoice is used to reach, inform, and organise community members, enabling them to prioritise their concerns and discuss problems and solutions. Photovoice goes beyond the conventional role of community assessment by inviting people to promote their own and their community's well-being. It is a method that enables people to define for themselves and others, including policy makers, what is worth remembering and what needs to be changed (Photovoice, 2008). Box 4.4 provides a case study example to illustrate how Photovoice can be used in a practical setting to address the issue of maternal and child health.

■ Health literacy

Health literacy is essentially a repackaging of the relationship between education and empowerment that has evolved as a concept within public health. It grew out of the realisation that interventions that relied heavily on information toward behaviour change failed to achieve substantial results and had little effect in closing the inequalities gap between different social and economic groups (Nutbeam, 2000). The unfulfilled potential of many education strategies in health promotion

Box 4.4 Photovoice for Maternal and Child Health

Contra Costa is a large, economically and ethnically diverse county in the San Francisco Bay area. Sixty county residents ages 13–50 participated in three sessions during which they received training from the local health department in the techniques and process of Photovoice. Residents were provided with disposable cameras and were encouraged to take photographs reflecting their views on family, maternal, and child health assets and concerns in their community, and then participated in group discussions about their photographs. Community events were held to enable participants to educate Maternal and Child Health (MCH) staff and community leaders.

Results: The Photovoice project provided MCH staff with information to supplement existing quantitative peri-natal data and contributed to an understanding of key MCH issues that participating community residents would like to see addressed. Participants concerns centred on the need for safe places for children's recreation and for improvement in the broader community environment within county neighbourhoods. Participants' definitions of family, maternal and child health assets and concerns differed from those that MCH professionals may typically view as MCH issues (low birth weight, maternal mortality, teen pregnancy prevention), which helped MCH program staff to expand priorities and include residents' foremost concerns.

Conclusions: MCH professionals can apply Photovoice as an innovative participatory research methodology to engage community members in needs assessment, asset mapping, and program planning, and in reaching policy makers to advocate strategies promoting family, maternal, and child health as informed from a grassroots perspective (Wang and Pies, 2004).

as a tool for social change and political action therefore left Practitioners searching for new alternatives.

What is new about health literacy is that health education becomes more than just the transmission of information and is focused on skills development and confidence building so as to help others to make better informed decisions that will allow them to gain greater control over their lives (Renkert and Nutbeam, 2001). Health literacy involves both cognitive and social skills which determine the motivation and ability of individuals to gain access to, understand and use information in ways that promote and maintain good health (WHO, 1998). Health literacy is dependent on the level of basic literacy in the community, that is, the ability to read and write in everyday life and what this enables people to do. Health literacy has three levels:

- *Basic/functional literacy* – sufficient basic skills in reading and writing to be able to function effectively in everyday situations, broadly compatible with the narrow definition.

- *Communicative/interactive literacy* – more advanced cognitive and literacy skills which, together with social skills, can be used to actively participate in everyday activities, to extract information and derive meaning from different forms of communication, and to apply new information to changing circumstances.
- *Critical literacy* – more advanced cognitive skills which, together with social skills, can be applied to critically analyse information, and to use this information to exert greater control over life events and situations (Nutbeam, 2000, p. 263).

The challenge in public health practice is to use advanced methods of health education aimed at achieving critical health literacy rather than basic or functional health literacy. The value of health literacy is therefore as a tool to help Practitioners to become more effective communicators by increasing the critical awareness of individual clients. The work of Paulo Freire, discussed earlier in Photovoice, has shown that working to raise the 'critical awareness' of people with poor basic literacy skills can lead to outcomes that are closely aligned with empowerment (Nutbeam, 2000). In a public health practice dominated by health education, health literacy offers an advance on this type of an approach that enables people to understand better the social determinants of their health and how to take action to address them. In Box 4.5 I provide the example of using health literacy to improve antenatal classes.

■ Fostering an empowering professional-client relationship

Fostering an empowering professional-client relationship describes a process in which power-over is used carefully and deliberately by the Practitioner to increase

---

Box 4.5 Health Literacy and Antenatal Classes

An example of the potential use of health literacy is for the development of antenatal classes to provide women with the cognitive and social skills to maintain their health and that of their children. Women attending antenatal classes are often highly motivated and literate. But antenatal classes are sometimes constrained by time and the natural curiosity and anxiety of the women makes it difficult to transfer all the necessary information and skills. Classes therefore focus on the transfer of factual information rather than on decision-making skills for childbirth and parenting which can occupy more time. The latter is empowering rather than just passive and central to the use of health literacy techniques that focuses on providing the necessary skills and enabling women to make informed choices. In this way the entire content of the antenatal class would not have to be delivered, reducing the time needed for teaching and providing more time to allow the mothers to ask questions and to discuss issues (Renkert and Nutbeam, 2001).

the power-from-within of their client. This is the transformative use of power-with as described in Chapter 2. The qualities of an empowering relationship include a non-coercive dialogue between the Practitioner and the client in the identification of problems and practical actions, such as developing a decision-making matrix (discussed earlier), to address and resolve problems. The key attributes of the Practitioner in an empowering role are as an 'enabler', facilitator, helper, counselor and guide. The purpose of the role is to use these attributes to support their clients to facilitate change in their lives through their own actions. The goal, for example, in the context of nursing care in a hospital was identified as enabling patients to take more control in decision making over their health, promoting patient independence, information exchange and being aware of their needs. In practice, this translated into acts of care such as making sure patients had their call bell within reach, respecting their choices, providing information about future care options and working quietly at night to allow patients to sleep (Faulkner, 2001).

However, not all Practitioners can apply an empowering approach to their everyday work, for example, those involved in enforcement, licensing and legal proceedings will have fewer opportunities to empower others than those professionals working in an advisory or counseling role with individuals. This is because enforcement uses a power-over approach to maintain authority in contrast to an advisory and educational role that can use a power-with approach to build the power-from-within of other people.

An empowering professional-client relationship involves many of the approaches and skills discussed in this book, for example, the ability to be a good communicator, a good listener, helping people to become more critically aware, dealing with conflict, linking individuals to groups that share interests and building the capacity of others. The language that we choose to use as professionals can have a significant influence upon the clients with whom we work. An empowering professional-client relationship in public health involves the Practitioner using an empowering discourse, ideology and language, that is conscious in linking the individual with the social and political context.

■ The power of language

Language exerts considerable force in our world constructions and this applies to our professional as well as our social worlds (Seidman and Wagner, 1992). In particular, the way in which 'to empower', the central action in an empowering public health practice, has been interpreted is critical. Labonte (1994, p. 255) discusses the transitive and intransitive meanings of the verb 'to empower'. The transitive (direct) meaning is to 'bestow power on others, an enabling act, sharing some of the power we hold over others'. Empowerment is cast as a relationship between the stakeholders of a programme, those with power-over and those without power. Empowerment becomes a dynamic in which this relationship continually shifts towards a more empowering situation where power is equitably shared between the stakeholders. However, the advantage is held by the one with the power-over and language becomes an important structuring factor in the professional-client relationship. The intransitive (indirect) meaning suggests the act of gaining or assuming power. This is the litmus test of empowerment because power in its purist form cannot be given but must be taken by individuals and groups who seek it. This is a process that can be facilitated by the Practitioner by helping to create the conditions necessary to make it possible for power to be gained. In a professional-client relationship, this is a mutual role played out by the Practitioner who facilitates change, and the client who identifies and executes the change. The language used in public health largely uses the meaning of both interpretations of power. But in practice, power cannot be given and clients must be enabled by Practitioners to gain or seize power from others. It is the relationship between the Practitioners and their clients that is therefore the mechanism to achieve greater control.

In public health practice, the advantage is often held by the one with the power over (the Practitioner) and the language that they choose to use can either strengthen or weaken the professional-client relationship. Box 4.6 shows how the use of language can have both an empowering and a non-empowering effect through the professional-client relationship. Both Accounts (1 and 2) are taken from the same case history file for Beatrice, an imaginary patient.

Box 4.6 Language and the Professional-Client Relationship

Which account of Beatrice is more empowering?

Account 1: Beatrice is

- a low income, single mother;
- unemployed;
- is undernourished and anaemic;
- is living in a one room basement apartment;
- looking after two children, her first child was of low birth weight;
- not able to speak English well;
- a smoker and drinks alcohol.

Account 2: Beatrice is

- looking for work that will fit her skills as a trained laboratory technician;
- is trying to find ways to supplement her diet but is unable to afford extra money for food shopping;
- living in a small tidy apartment but is looking for better accommodation;
- looking after her two healthy and happy children;
- learning English at night-class but finds it difficult to get a baby sitter;
- fluent in Spanish and French;
- trying to give up smoking.

Adapted from Labonte, 1998, p. 46.

The first account of Beatrice uses a power over approach in which the Practitioner presents a series of negative statements about the client, for example, Beatrice is described as being 'unemployed', 'undernourished' and having 'a low birth weight' child. The first account implies a person who is unhealthy and powerless and when confronted by such a description, through her contact with different Practitioners and institutions, Beatrice may begin to internalise it as being true about herself. This process is called learned helplessness, discussed in Chapter 2, and is a manifestation of power-over the client by the Practitioners or by the agency with which they work.

In the second account of Beatrice she is portrayed by using positive language centred around her own capacities or power-base, for example, 'trying to give up smoking', 'fluent in French and Spanish' and 'trained laboratory technician'. The account implies that the client is struggling but at the same time is trying to help herself and her family. It is a manifestation of power-from-within by the client and offers opportunities to develop an empowering professional-client relationship.

However, in a public health system that is sensitive to the poor and vulnerable people in society the negative description of Beatrice (Account 1) may actually be more empowering. The system is designed to respond to Beatrice's needs and provides her with support from social and welfare services to, for example, find employment, childcare and better housing. The positive description of Beatrice (Account 2) on the other hand may result in her needs being overlooked by the public health system as she is judged as not being vulnerable or at any immediate risk.

Technical terms are a part of the everyday language of Practitioners, for example, medical diagnostic vocabulary, and have evolved as knowledge and skills develop within a profession's 'subculture' (other subcultures include ethnic groups, social class, sexuality). However the use of specialist language is often confusing to lay people or to professionals not part of the 'subculture'. This can contribute to their sense of powerlessness by emphasising a lack of access to knowledge and the 'expert' power of the other person using the language. The use of terms such as 'high risk' and 'target group' imply passivity and locate the problem within the group rather than as a relationship to the broader social and environmental health determinants. Whilst it may sometimes be necessary to use specific technical terms the professional-client relationship is more empowering when it uses language and terminology that is understood by the receivers so that they are not confused, alienated or mystified by the communicator. To build the power-from-within of their clients the Practitioner must relinquish the control over the use of technical language and engage in a more empowering language.

What an empowering professional language means in practice is that the Practitioners should be aware that no discourse is value-free. It is important to understand the influence of their professional language and to be sensitive to the position and perceptions of their individual clients. Such awareness is termed a 'reflexive practice' in which the Practitioners are critical about the way they use their knowledge and power to have professional influence over other professionals and their clients. Scrambler (1987) provides an example of a consultation between a health professional and the client, a pregnant woman. The Practitioner began the discussion using 'lay' terms to describe the complications associated with her condition but quickly switched to a technical-rational language when her advice was challenged by the client. The client was then coerced into complying with the Practitioner because she suddenly felt uncertain and lacking in knowledge. The client had been dis-empowered by the Practitioner who was unaware of the switch to a technical, power-over use of language.

Next, Chapter 5 discusses how Practitioners, in their everyday work, can help groups and communities to gain power and introduces a framework that strengthens the capacity of people to better organise and mobilise themselves.

Chapter 5

Helping groups and communities to gain power

Helping groups and communities to gain power involves capacity building and community action. But to understand how a more empowering approach to public health practice can be applied in a collective context it is first important to consider what a 'community' is.

■ What is a 'community'?

It is important for Practitioners to think beyond the customary view of a community as a place where people live such as a village or neighbourhood because such areas can be just an aggregate of non-connected people. The fundamental issue when working with communities is whether they are social or geographic. Jim Ward, a Practitioner with experience of working with 'street communities' in Brisbane, Sydney and Toronto, describes these as 'groups of people perceiving common needs and problems, that acquire a sense of identity focussed around these problems and that a common set of objectives grow out of these identified issues' (Ward, 1987, p. 18). What can be concluded is that geographic communities consist of heterogeneous individuals with changing and dynamic social relations who may organise into groups to take action towards achieving shared goals. The concept of 'community' includes several key characteristics and these have been listed in Box 5.1.

Box 5.1   The Key Characteristics of 'Community'

1. A spatial dimension, that is, a place or locale.
2. Non-spatial dimensions (interests, issues, identities) that involve people who otherwise make up heterogeneous and disparate groups.
3. Social interactions that are dynamic and bind people into relationships with one another.
4. Identification of shared needs and concerns that can be achieved through a process of collective action.

Adapted from Laverack, 2004, p. 46.

The diversity of individuals and groups within a geographic community can create problems with regard to the selection of representation by its members (Zakus and Lysack, 1998). Practitioners need to carefully consider who the legitimate representatives of a community are. Those individuals who have the energy, time and motivation to become involved in activities may, in fact, not be supported by other community members and may be considered as acting out of self-interest. In these circumstances, a dominant minority may dictate the community needs unless adequate actions are taken to involve everyone.

Within the geographic or spatial dimensions of a 'community', multiple communities can exist and individuals may belong to several different 'interest' groups or communities at the same time. Interest groups exist as a legitimate means by which individuals can find a 'voice' and are able to participate in a more formal way to achieve their goals, for example, through committees, social clubs and religious associations. Interest groups provide the opportunity for people to collectively address mutual concerns, for example, the members of a smoking cessation club or people who have concerns about the siting of a new airport. A group setting provides individuals with a means through which they can take a step closer towards achieving their goals. This involves the collective action of individuals who share the same concerns and form a 'community of interest' which in turn seeks to gain more control over resources and decisions. This process is called 'community empowerment'.

■ Community empowerment as a 5-point continuum

Community empowerment has been most consistently viewed in the literature as a 5-point continuum comprised of the following elements:

Figure 5.1   The continuum of community empowerment

★	★	★	★	★
Personal action	Small groups	Community organisations	Partnerships	Social and political action

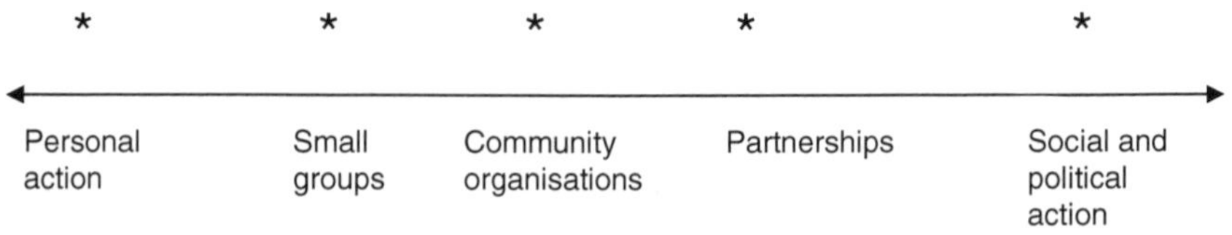

Adapted from Laverack, 1999, p. 92.

Labonte (1990) claims that the continuum was first developed in Australia in workshops with health and social service workers in 1988. Labonte subsequently published his version of the continuum for community empowerment followed by Jackson et al. (1989) who published their version for community development in 1989 using a similar 5-point continuum. Rissel (1994) later adapted these two interpretations of the continuum to explain how psychological empowerment relates to the process of community empowerment. These three authors use slightly different terminologies that essentially hold the same meaning and represent the same conceptual design: the potential of people to progress from individual to collective action along a continuum.

The continuum model has remained unchallenged in the literature and explains how collective action can potentially be maximised as people progress from individual to community empowerment. The continuum model offers a simple, linear interpretation of what is actually a dynamic and complex concept. The continuum also articulates the various levels of empowerment from personal, to organisational through collective (community) action. Each point on the continuum can be viewed as a progression towards the goal of community empowerment. If a way forward is not possible stasis occurs or a move back to the preceding point on the continuum.

The development of a community organisation on the continuum is pivotal to allow small groups to make the transition to a broader network of alliances. It is through these partnerships that organisations are able to gain greater support and resources to achieve a favourable outcome for their particular concerns. The key challenge to public health is how Practitioners and the agencies they represent structure their work with the explicit intent to assist individuals and groups in their progression along the continuum.

There are limitations to the concept of a continuum of community empowerment because the groups and organisations that arise have their own dynamics. They may flourish for a time, then fade away for reasons as much to do with changes in the people and community as with a lack of broader political or financial support. Public health practice is a part of this dynamic, an important part that, as I explain in this book, can help people to become more empowered.

■ The 'domains' of community empowerment

Several authors have attempted to identify the areas of influence on community empowerment (Goodman et al., 1998; Laverack, 2001; Rifkin et al., 1988). In Table 5.1, I summarise the work of other authors to identify the areas of influence of overlapping concepts with community empowerment. This work has assisted in the identification of both social and organisational aspects and has been a useful step towards making this complex concept more operational. The practical purpose is to provide a guide to Practitioners in their planning, application and evaluation of empowerment approaches in public health programmes.

Laverack (2001) identified a set of nine 'domains' of community empowerment through a review of relevant literature, with particular reference to the fields of health, social sciences and education. This provided an in-depth understanding of programmes which sought to achieve the same empowerment goals: to bring about social and political change. Laverack's 'domains' were categorised from a textual analysis of the literature and the validity of this data was cross-checked by

Table 5.1 The overlap of empowering concepts (from Laverack, 2001)

Community participation Ritkin (1988) Factors	Community competence Eng and Parker (1994)	Community participation Shrimpton (1995) Indicators	Community empowerment domains Laverack (2001) Dimensions	Community capacity Goodman et al. (1998) Dimensions
	Participation, machinery for participant interaction and decision making		Participation	Participation
Leadership		Leadership	Leadership	Leadership
Organisation	Social support	Organisation	Organisational structures	Sense of community, an understanding of community history and values
Resource Mobilisation		Resource Mobilisation	Resource Mobilisation	Resources
Needs Assessment		Needs Assessment/ action choice	Problem assessment	
	Self aware, clarity of definitions		Asking why	Critical reflection
	Management of relations with wider society		Links with others	Social and inter-organisational networks
			Outside agents	
Management-programme	Conflict containment	Management (programme)	Programme management	Skills
	Articulation	Training		Community power
	Commitment	Orientation of actions		
		Monitoring and evaluation		

two other researchers using a confusion matrix approach as discussed by Robson (1993, p. 222).

1. Community participation;
2. Problem assessment capacities;
3. Local leadership;
4. Organisational structures;
5. Resource mobilisation;
6. Links to other organisations and people;
7. Ability to 'ask why' (critical awareness);
8. Community control over programme management; and
9. An equitable relationship with outside agents.

Table 5.2 The empowerment domains (Laverack and Labonte, 2000)

Domain	Description
Participation	Only by participating in small groups or larger organisations can individual community members act on issues of general concern to the broader community.
Leadership	Participation and leadership are closely connected. Leadership requires a strong participant base just as participation requires the direction and structure of strong leadership.
Organisational structures	Organisational structures in a community represent the ways in which people come together in order to socialise and to address their concerns and problems.
Problem assessment	Empowerment presumes that the identification of problems, solutions to the problems and actions to resolve the problems are carried out by the community.
Resource mobilisation	The ability of the community to mobilise resources both from within and the ability to negotiate resources from beyond itself is an important factor in its ability so achieve successes in its efforts.
'Asking why'	The ability of the community to critically assess the causes of its own inequalities.
Links with others	Links with people and organisations, including partnerships, coalitions and voluntary alliances between the community and others, can assist the community in addressing its issues.
Role of the outside agents	The outside agent increasingly transforms power relationships such that the community assumes increasing programme authority.
Programme management	Programme management that empowers the community includes the control by the primary stakeholders over decisions on planning, implementation, evaluation, finances, reporting and conflict resolution.

A description of each domain is given in Table 5.2. Laverack's 'domains approach' has proved robust across a range of settings and has been successfully extended to provide a guide for health programming and measurement. Examples of its application are discussed in detail in Chapters 6 and 7.

A 'domains approach' gives a more precise way of developing empowerment strategies whilst at the same time helping to progress people along the continuum in Figure 5.1. The key question Practitioners need to ask themselves is: How has the programme, from its planning through its implementation, through its evaluation, intentionally sought to enhance community empowerment in each domain? (Laverack, 2004). I will now discuss a framework to explain how Practitioners can build more empowered groups and communities and relate this to the theory on the continuum model and 'domains' approach for empowerment, discussed earlier.

■ A framework for helping groups and communities to gain power

The role of the Practitioner when using this framework increasingly becomes that of an enabler, at the request of the clients, to provide resources, services and information. Table 5.3 summarises the key enabling roles of the Practitioner in the community empowerment continuum model. The basic logic offered by the framework can be seen in everyday life by groups and communities seeking to

Table 5.3 Key enabling roles in the continuum model

Continuum model	Key role of the Practitioner
Personal action	Build a greater sense of control in peoples' lives and bring them together in small groups around issues of mutual concern.
Small mutual groups	Assist the community to identify and prioritise its problems, solutions to the problems and actions to resolve the problems. To strengthen local leadership skills.
Community organisations	Strengthen organisational structures. Link organisations to resources and develop skills to identify, mobilise and access resources. Promote critical awareness.
Partnerships	To develop a shared agenda with other organisations and build local partnerships and alliances between groups. Provide access to resources outside the community.
Social and political action	Provide legitimacy to the issues and concerns raised by the community by using their own expert power and political influence.

gain power. This is often voiced as a struggle for social justice and equity, for example, the localised actions of residents to gain adequate street lighting or the wider actions of citizens publically demonstrating against what they see as poor governance in their country.

■ Empowering individuals for personal action

A personal action to improve health can begin when individuals feel powerless about a situation, feel the desire to rectify, what they perceive as, an unjust situation or want to take action in response to an emotive experience in their lives. Kieffer (1984) provides an example of how this happened to one woman who became active in a small community support group for neighbourhood safety following an assault on her way home from work one evening. The self-help group she joined was working towards addressing the issues of her concern, for example, improved policing and public transport in her neighbourhood. In a programme context, the basis for personal action is most often developed during the planning phase through an identification of participants' problems and later developed as a part of the objectives.

Individuals have a better chance of achieving their goals if they can share their concern with other people who are affected by the same or similar circumstances. By participating in groups and organisations, individuals can better define, analyse and then, through the support of others, act on their concerns. Zakus and Lysack (1998, p. 2) provide a useful definition of participation set in this context as 'the process by which members of the community, either individually or collectively and with varying degrees of commitment: develop the capability to assume greater responsibility for assessing their health needs and problems; plan and then act to implement their solutions and create and maintain organisations in support of these efforts'.

However, research in the UK has shown that of 55% of local residents who said they wanted to participate in a programme in regard to a road that was being built through their community, only 2% actually did participate (CBI, 2006, p. 2). Engaging with community members to ensure that they fully participate in programmes can be a crucial factor for success or failure.

Bracht and Tsouros (1990) and Goodman et al. (1998) address the issue of how individuals participate and agree in their conclusions that it is a combination of involvement in decision-making mechanisms, accessibility to community organisations and the development of appropriate skills such as planning and resource mobilisation. The advantage of participation is that community-based organisations are better at strengthening social networks, competing for limited resources and increasing the necessary skills and competencies of its members. Empowering individuals for action must therefore involve helping them to participate in group and community activities.

Box 5.2 provides some of the main characteristics of participation in empowering others for personal action.

Box 5.2 The Characteristics of Participation in Empowering Others

1. A strong participant base involving all stakeholders, including marginalised groups, but sensitive to the cultural and social context.
2. Participants define their own needs, solutions and actions.
3. Participants involved in decision-making mechanisms at planning, implementation and evaluation stages.
4. Participants are encouraged to extend into broader issues of the structural causes of powerlessness and to become critically self-aware.
5. Mechanisms exist to allow free flow of information between the different participants through effective communication.
6. Representatives are appointed by members of all groups.
7. The Practitioner fosters an empowering professional-client relationship.
Adapted from Laverack, 1999.

■ Empowering small groups

The involvement in and the development of small groups by concerned individuals is the start of collective action. This locale provides an opportunity for the Practitioner to assist the individual to gain skills and to link them to groups and organisations that develop stronger social support and that mobilise the resources necessary to support collective action.

Small 'interest' groups include:

1. 'Self-help' or 'interest' groups organised around a specific problem such as 'Weight Watchers' or consumers wanting to find suppliers for organically grown produce. Members usually have a shared knowledge and interest in the problem, are participatory and supportive and the groups are often set-up and managed by the participants;
2. Community health groups that usually come together to campaign on a specific issue, for example, facilities for socially excluded groups such as the elderly. People are motivated to come together usually for short-term periods of time, however, these groups can also form long-lasting associations such as NIMBY's (Not In My Back Yard) in regard to broader issues that influence geographical community such as the siting of a radio mast; and
3. Community development health projects such as neighbourhood-based projects set up to address issues of local concern such as poor housing, and with an appointed and paid government community worker (discussed further in Jones and Sidell, 1997).

The role of the Practitioner at this point of the continuum is to bring people together and to help them, through a range of participatory techniques, to identify issues which they feel are important to them. Problem assessment skills are necessary for small groups to be able to identify the common problems of their members, solutions to the problems and actions to resolve the problems. When these skills do not exist or are weak the role of the Practitioner will be to assist the community to make an assessment of its own problems. A number of participatory methods have been developed specifically for this purpose including Participatory Rural Appraisal (Marsden et al., 1994) and I discuss problem assessment in Chapter 3.

Andrew Jones and Glenn Laverack (2003) identify a number of characteristics of small, functional and successful 'interest' groups:

- Had a membership of elected representatives;
- The majority of its members met on a regular basis;
- Had an agreed membership structure (chairperson, secretary, core members, etc.);
- All members actively participated in the meetings;
- The group met with a Practitioner to discuss issues on a regular basis;
- Kept records of previous meetings;
- Kept financial accounts;
- Were able to identify and resolve conflicts quickly; and
- Were able to identify the 'problems' of and the resources available to the 'interest group'.

Each group they observed had achieved a number of goals, such as repairs to a school roof, better access to quality agricultural products or improvements to an irrigation system. These small successes had helped to build the confidence and the connectedness of the members of the group. However, not all groups were found to be functional and those that were not successful showed the characteristics of a limited capacity, for example, a focus on immediate problems often viewed by the group as important issues without longer-term planning. Consequently, the less functional groups viewed Practitioners not as partners in helping them to build their own capacity but rather as sources of credit (the term 'partner' implies a working relationship based on recognition of overlapping or mutual interests, and interpersonal and inter-organisational respect). The Practitioners were unintentionally acting as top-down and power-over sources of assistance even though their purpose was to facilitate a bottom-up and power-with approach (Jones and Laverack, 2003).

Small 'interest' groups have limited resources and because of their size the inclusion in the policy process can actually lead to them being absorbed whilst at the same time adding legitimacy to governments who pursue a larger agenda. Their low level of participation and poor resource base provide them with little influence (Allsop, Jones and Baggott, 2004). To have more influence the small groups need to grow and develop into broader community-based organisations.

■ Empowering groups to develop into community organisations

Community organisations include committees, co-operatives and associations. These are the organisational elements in which people come together in order to socialise and to take action to address their broader concerns. Community organisations are not only larger than small groups they also have an established structure, more functional leadership, the ability to better organise their members to mobilise resources and to gain the skills that are necessary to make the transition to partnerships and alliances. These skills include planning and strategy development, management of time, team building, networking, negotiation, fund-raising, marketing, managing publicity and proposal writing. While small groups generally focus inwards on the needs of their members, community organisations focus outwards to the environment that creates those needs in the first place, or offers the means (resources, opportunities) to resolving them. Once the community has become more critically aware of the underlying causes of its powerlessness they can then take the necessary steps to develop actions to redress the situation and to try to gain more power for themselves.

Community organisations enable people to progress along the empowerment continuum by improving the ability of small groups to access internal and external resources. Internal resources are those raised within the community and include land, food, money, people skills and local knowledge. External resources are those brought into the community by, for example, the Practitioner, and include financial assistance, technical expertise, 'new' knowledge and equipment. The ability of the community to mobilise resources from within and to negotiate resources from beyond itself is an indication of a high degree of skill and organisation. The role of the Practitioner is that of a link between appropriate resource

---

Box 5.3 The 'Toilet Festivals' of Mumbai, India

Community-based organisations set up in the slums of Mumbai, India identified the problem of poor sanitation and water supply as a key concern to the residents. The organisations developed a strategy to host 'toilet festivals' as official opening ceremonies for sanitary facilities in the community. The press were invited and the usual protocol for a ceremony was held with guests invited to attend and banners advertising the event posted. The real purpose of the 'toilet festivals' was to engage with municipal officials firstly by demonstrating the initiative of slum dwellers to organise their own construction of sanitary facilities but secondly to draw the officials into the debate about the lack of resources and infra-structure. The agenda was re-orientated to include poor living conditions and not solely the previous focus of illegal settlement. The media was able to raise the issue and the slum dwellers were able to short-cut the normal channels of bureaucracy and power-over structures in local government (Appadurai, 2004).

sources and the community organisation and to find creative ways to communicate their ideas and to express themselves. An example of this is in Box 5.3 of
'Toilet Festivals' of Mumbai, India in which settlement dwellers organised themselves into organisations and used their resources to draw municipal officials into
negotiations.

The development of community organisations and local leadership are closely
connected. Leadership requires a strong participant base just as community
organisations require the direction and structure of strong leadership (Goodman
et al., 1998). Anderson, Shepard, and Salisbury (2006) found that exceptional
local people who had a shared commitment to public involvement were important
to motivate others in the community and to develop partnerships. Local people
were drawn into the process of participation and with increased confidence and
capacity became powerful advocates for their community. A proper balance
between professional inputs and lay people was seen as essential because conflict
was found to occur over the lack of clarity of who has control in the programme.
When leaders appear to have a limited vision of their aims or lack a strategy, the
role of the Practitioner is to help develop their skills, for example, in management,
accounting and proposal writing.

The Practitioner should carefully consider: who represents the 'community',
how they are selected, what is their existing level of training and skills and what is
the balance between their economic and traditional influence in the community?
The problem of selecting appropriate leadership is discussed by Goodman et al.
(1998), who argue that a pluralistic approach in the community, one where there

---

Box 5.4 Misrepresentation by Local Leadership

Lucy Earle et al. (2004, p. 27), a community development researcher, and
her colleagues provide an example of the manipulation of programmes by
local leaders in Central Asia. The village leader in one community had used
his influence to obtain assistance from an NGO to help provide irrigation
pipes and an electric pump to improve the water supply of the community.
But not all members of the community were satisfied with these develop-
ments, especially groups of low-income women. The water supplied was too
expensive for them and the pipes were laid to better serve the family members of the village leader. However, they could not complain because to contradict the leader could mean serious consequences for the livelihoods of
poor families; for example, the village leader provided temporary employment during harvest and distributed flour to poorer residents. Not only did
the leader hold an influential position in the community but his sons also
held posts in the local government administration. The village leader was
able to use his power-over others in the community, mostly over marginalised groups, to manipulate the distribution of resources and gain access to
decision-making processes.

is an interplay between the positional leaders, those who have been elected or appointed and the reputed leaders, those who informally serve the community, has a better chance of leading to community empowerment. Otherwise, the dominance of one leader may result in them using their power-over the community, or groups within the community, to manipulate situations to their own advantage. To illustrate this Box 5.4 provides an example of how local leaders can misrepresent the interests of their community.

■ Empowering community organisations to develop partnerships

To be effective in influencing 'higher level' decision making, community organisations need to link with others sharing similar concerns. The purpose of partnerships is to allow community organisations to grow beyond their own local concerns and to take a stronger position on broader issues through networking and resource mobilisation. The key empowerment issue is to remain focused on the shared concern that brings the groups together, and not on the individual

---

Box 5.5 Cluster Communities as Partnerships in North America

Korsching and Borich (1997, p. 342) provide a useful account in Iowa, America of how rural communities started to empower themselves by forming clusters. A cluster community is defined as 'voluntary alliances between two or more communities to address common problems, needs and interests'. The communities were faced with concerns common to many rural populations: a lack of resources; a decline in employment; loss of young people and the closing of businesses and institutions caused by sweeping social and economic changes in society. In response, many community groups adopted a similar strategy of creating partnerships to pool resources, discuss issues and plan for action. Korsching and Borich (1997) argue that the emergence of cluster communities follows a familiar pattern; initiation by a concerned individual or organisation, establishment of meetings with other groups, formal organisation, development of further links and partnerships through an expansion of community concerns to address broader issues. To be successful, the clusters initially remained small scale but soon became legal entities and developed links with private and public organisations such as companies and universities. The strength of the cluster concept lies in its ability to establish productive links with others whilst at the same time remaining flexible and small enough to allow the participation of community members to be maintained. The role of the Practitioner was first to help to bring cluster communities together and then to support the positions raised by local partnerships, helping to legitimise the issues by their 'expert' power in the development of supporting policy.

needs of the different groups in the partnership. Box 5.5 provides an example of how small rural communities in Iowa, America started to empower themselves by forming cluster communities around shared needs.

Partnerships that place an emphasis on public involvement, especially in deprived areas have had some success (Anderson et al., 2006) such as the Health Park concept in the UK that was a joint venture of government, private and public interests. Other partnerships in the UK such as the national lottery can also be a means to promote flexible funding and innovative collaborations towards empowerment.

■ Empowering communities to take social and political action

Whilst individuals are able to influence the direction and implementation of a programme through their participation this alone does not constitute community empowerment. If concerned individuals remained at the small group level, the conditions leading to their powerlessness would not be resolved. Equally, if concerned individuals only engaged in mainstream forms of 'action' such as voting, when their concerns are often diluted by being represented by people in authority and by decisions being made centrally, those with power-over economic and political decisions would have little reason to listen. The individual plays a small part in the process and his/her role is often indirect and passive, for example, writing to a local political representative, registering a complaint or signing a petition.

Practitioners are involved in approaches in their day-to-day work in ways that can help their clients to become more critically aware and to take a more active role in social and political issues through collective action. This involves encouraging their participation in community groups and organisations and in partnership development towards direct actions such as publicity campaigns, civil protests, public demonstrations and legal action, discussed in Chapter 2.

Gaining power to influence economic, political, social and ideological change will inevitably involve the individuals, groups and communities in a struggle with those already holding power. Within a programme context the traditional role of the Practitioner is to build capacity, provide resources and technical support. But Practitioners need to recognise that an empowering public health practice is a political activity. The structures of power-over, of bureaucracy and authority remain dominant and their role, at least in part, is to strive to challenge these circumstances.

Finally, it is important to recognise that empowerment takes on meaning in relation to issues around which the group impetus grows or fades. There is never absolute power or empowerment for individuals, groups and communities. Rather, both only ever exist in relation to particular issues around which clients act together to create, or to resist, change. It is through individual action and collective empowerment that people can gain the power that is necessary to address their concerns. The skills, competencies and capacities that they will need to develop can be supported as part of the everyday work of Practitioners. The framework discussed in this chapter is a means to better conceptualise how individuals can progress from a position of personal concern to a point where they are collectively and actively involved with redressing the deeper underlying causes that influence peoples' health and lives, such as, poverty, unemployment and powerlessness.

Social movements can provide an important partnership for community-based organisations that are searching for wider social and political action, participation and the access to resources. They also provide a bridge between the ideology that many community-based organisations espouse on empowerment, emancipation and liberation and the established discourse.

■ Social movements

Although there is no real agreement as to the nature of social movements one major division has been between the views of structural conflict and those that interpret movements as a normal part of change in society. The diversity of the interpretations of social movements to some extent mirrors the diversity of theoretical and ideological allegiances. In recent years social movements have popularly been viewed by scholars in Westernised countries along three schema; Resource Mobilisation Theory (RMT), popular with American researchers taking an economic rationalism view, Action Identity Theory (AIT) and New Social Movement Theory (NSMT) popular with European researchers and based on Marxist and Durkheimian traditions. It is the emancipatory discourse of the NSMT that is shared by what has been termed the 'new public health movement' (Baum, 1990). However, this term can be misleading because it hides the bureaucratic and sometimes controlling nature of public health towards civil society. Social movements have a structure, a pattern of inter-relations between individuals and groups. This pattern evolves through its processes of mobilisation, participation and organisation. Formal social movements may possess bureaucratic procedures but they do not operate from within bureaucracies. Social movements exist within civil society as community-based groups, developed by the people, against systematic structures and ideologies held by those in authority (Pakulski, 1991).

A distinction can also be made between what are considered to be 'old' social movements and 'new' social movements (Melucci, 1985). New social movements are not solely concerned with structural revolution or reform but more with cultural and expressive objectives based on the formation of an identity. Identity is created not simply through the existence of a social movement but through action within the movement. The identity is shared by all its members and it is the process of internal action and negotiation that connects and bonds them through social relationships. The main purpose of the 'new' movements is their transformation of values and change, for example, in the nature of health care and social services, rather than a radical restructuring. In the context of 'new' public health movements the process and outcome of such action is to promote the health and well-being of its members. For example, the collective action among mental health service users in Nottingham in England who formed the Nottingham

Advocacy Group. This group grew out of the meetings held by patients on hospital wards and with the support of similar groups slowly developed into a national advisory network. Whilst involved in the personal development of its members the main aim of the group was to have an influence on shaping mental health policy and services (Barnes, 2002).

In particular, new social movement 'Health Social Movements' (HSMs) are an important point of social interaction concerning the rights of people to access health services, personal experiences of illness, disease and disability and health inequality based on race, class, gender and sexuality. The growing awareness of health science that has become available through, for example, the internet, has led to people challenging public health policy. This has been coupled by the negative publicity received about bio-medical abuses of authority such as experimentation with contraceptives, radiation and immunisation that has created a heightened level of distrust by the public toward, in particular, the medical profession. People have discovered that collectively they can apply significant pressure to influence public policy that affects their health at an individual level (Brown and Zavestoski, 2004). HSMs ultimately challenge state, institutional and other forms of authority to give the public more of a voice in public health policy and regulation. HSMs overlap in their purpose and tactics but can be categorised into three ideal types (Brown et al., 2004, pp. 685–6):

1. Health access movements that seek equitable access to health care services, for example, through national health care reforms and an extension of health insurance to non-insured sectors of the population;
2. Embodied health movements concern people who want to address personal experiences of disease, illness and disability through a challenge of the scientific evidence by medical recognition of their ideas or their own research. It can include people directly affected by a condition or those who feel they are an at risk group, for example, the AIDS movement.
3. Constituency-based health movements concern health inequalities when the evidence shows an oversight or disproportionate outcome and include the homosexual movements and environmental rights.

HSMs are clearly not the sole source of health policy change but they can play and important role, one that is sometimes undervalued, and Box 5.6 provides an example of the actions of an important HSM: the environmental breast cancer movement.

HSMs have been effective in influencing other movements and public health policy by changing individuals and the values that they hold. This links into the work by Ron Eyerman, a sociologist, and Andrew Jamison, an academic interested in social and political policy (1991). These researchers add to the discussion on social movements by examining their intellectual and political activities. Eyerman and Jamison argue that these activities can change societal values and norms, for example, public values towards health issues such as smoking and air pollution. In particular, there are two main concepts in the approaches that they

Box 5.6   The Environmental Breast Cancer Movement in the USA

The environmental breast cancer movement in the US was formed by a spill-over from the women's movement, AIDS activism and the environmental movements that created a HSM able to identify with those at risk from or affected by breast cancer. Maren Klawiter (2004, pp. 865–6) discusses the early experiences of women in the 1970s in the San Francisco Bay Area with breast cancer who endured isolation, power inequalities structured around the doctor-patient relationship and gender. The breast cancer movement provided many people with the intellectual and emotional support they needed to be able to move forward collectively to address a personal issue. Using the lessons that they had brought with them they pressed for expanded clinical trials, compassionate access to new drugs and greater government funding. HSMs use other tactics such as engaging in legal action, support to new research, creative media campaigns and influencing the policy process (Brown and Zavestoski, 2004). Twenty years later a new regime of breast cancer had emerged influenced by the efforts of the environmental breast cancer movement. Women had access to feminist and gay friendly cancer centres, patient education workshops, support groups, a choice of medical alternatives and a role as part of the health care team that delivered the cancer treatment. Essentially, breast cancer had become politicised and reframed as a feminist issue and an environmental disease.

discuss that are relevant to the evolution of empowerment in public health discourse: cognitive praxis; and movement intellectuals.

Cognitive praxis is the 'knowledge interests' that are held by a movement and the 'dynamic and mediating role that movements play in the shaping of knowledge' (Eyerman and Jamison, 1991, p. 47). This is the origin of new knowledge generated by a movement and 'intellectuals' within the movement draw upon and reinterpret established intellectual concepts. Cognitive praxis plays another important role, the development of new societal images and identities. Examples of how society transforms its self-identity through the knowledge generated by social movements include setting new problems for society to solve and advancing new values for ethical identification by individuals.

Eyerman and Jamison identify that the role of movement actors is normally viewed as those that lead and those that are led, and that the role of 'movement intellectuals' to strategically plan and create new knowledge is an important one which is often overlooked. As the movement matures and new organisations emerge there may be a transformation in the relationship between the intellectual and the movement. Movement intellectuals occupy the 'space' created for them temporarily before they seek legitimacy elsewhere, for example, in academia, media and government agencies. They establish their new identities and thus act as a vehicle through which movement knowledge can be dispersed socially. In this way, intellectuals create movements and movements create intellectuals in processes within society to challenge conventional knowledge and wisdom. Eyerman and Jamison (1991) theorise that movements are the engines of social change and contribute in this way to contemporary discourse. As the movements create new knowledge and intellectuals both become absorbed and institutionalised by society they create a bridge between new knowledge challenges and the established knowledge constructions and practice.

In this way the legitimisation of the discourse on public health issues has been influenced through the absorption of movement 'intellectuals' either into, or their direct influence upon government, academic and private sector agencies. In particular, the main themes of the discourse of NSMT, emancipation, inequality, and social justice, based on the evidence from the research or personal experience has relevance to an empowering public health practice. Movements have an emancipatory role and place an emphasis on challenges to counter authoritative forms of power-over and the dominant discourse that has been taken for granted, created whilst gaining political legitimacy (Eyerman and Jamison, 1991).

Public health itself is not a social movement because whilst it may share an emancipatory discourse, in practice it is carried out within the controlling sphere of bureaucratic settings. Public health remains disease-based, embracing a biomedical interpretation of health and employing top-down approaches to programming. Its purpose is to reduce the burden of disease and programme goals remain driven by the reduction of morbidity and mortality. This bureaucratic logic can prevent Practitioners from employing and their clients from engaging with empowerment approaches.

Next, in Chapter 6, I discuss the means by which Practitioners can help marginalised people to gain power and, in particular, discuss examples of helping to empower indigenous and migrant communities involved in public health programmes.

Chapter 6

Helping marginalised people to gain power

■ Marginalisation

Marginalisation is a process by which an individual or a group of individuals are denied access to, or positions of, for example, economic, religious and political power within a society (Marshall, 1998). Marginalisation is relevant to public health practice because these groups often exist on the fringes of a society from where they can become excluded from access to health services. It is a paradox of empowerment approaches that the most marginalised people are often unable to articulate their needs, are not represented or are unaware of opportunities and, as a result, do not have the opportunity to voice their concerns. The circumstances of their marginalisation, or the low self-esteem that it produces, can also contribute to their exclusion from, for example, main stream public health programming.

In practical terms marginalised groups are considered to be those that are most in need, not able to meet their own needs, have a limited access to resources, are powerless or exist largely outside dominant social power structures. Marginalised groups include the elderly, the mentally ill and people of a low socio-economic status such as migrant workers. But marginalisation can also be based on gender, ethnicity, (dis)ability and sexual preference. Although marginal groups are often a small population size relative to other groups in society they can actually be a numerical majority, for example, coloured people in South Africa during apartheid. Simpson and Yinger (1965) provide a broad-based interpretation that does not place a numerical value on minority but its emphasis is on the social position of the group:

> Minorities are subordinate segments of complex state societies, have special physical or cultural traits that are held in low esteem by the dominant segments of the society, are self-conscious units bound together by special traits which their members share (Simpson and Yinger, 1965, p. 17).

This definition also refers to the psychological status of the minority and their status within social power structures: do they feel themselves to be members of a particular social group that is clearly distinguished by them from other such groups? The group regard themselves as objects of collective discrimination having been singled out from the majority of others in the society in which they live, or by those who hold positions of power, for unequal treatment.

Practitioners who want to work with marginalised groups must have a clear understanding of the circumstances that cause the marginalisation of their clients, for example, inequalities in access to services, prejudicial policies, negative societal attitudes or hegemonic power structures that can exclude those who do not conform to societal values.

Ideally, Practitioners work with those in greatest need and strive to avoid the establishment of a dominant minority that might dictate community issues and marginalise people. This requires some judgement on the part of the Practitioner that people coming forward as representatives of a community are in fact supported by its members and have their best interest at heart. Box 6.1 is an attempt to define more specifically some of the criteria for selecting and working with groups, based on the principles of empowerment and social justice.

Box 6.1   Criteria for Selecting Community Groups

1. **The group has unmet needs**
   - the unorganised
   - groups that are neglected by other service providers, politicians, the media
   - groups experiencing serious disadvantages
   - groups who don't know how to 'use' the 'system'

2. **Our support will have an impact**
   - the group is able to identify its goals and objectives and to focus on an issue
   - the group become able to organise itself and its own activities, and to act upon its issue
   - leadership arises within the group
   - there is a sufficient membership within the groups that some success will be likely
   - the group is able to achieve some short-term, visible successes
   - there is a sizeable number of people whose health will be affected positively by the group's success

3. **A new group needs to be organised**
   - there are no other agencies better able to do the organising
   - there is a critical mass of individuals who express interest in meeting as a group
   - there is health institution support and clear decision making to do the organising
   - there is positive movement in group dynamics; the group will not become stuck in an unproductive rut
   - the group develops a sense of responsibility for its own actions

Box 6.1   Criteria for Selecting Community Groups – *continued*

4. **I have knowledge or skills relevant to the group's issue**

5. **The group will grow and become autonomous**
    - the group knows or learns its rights, privileges and responsibilities
    - the group is or can become independent of the health promoter and community agencies, able to negotiate its own terms of relationships with those workers and agencies
    - the group learns how to look for, and use, resources from within its own community, and from government

6. **The group is open in membership and accountable to those it claims to represent**
    Groups might be inclusive (open to anyone who wants to join) or exclusive (closed except to those who meet its own criteria, e.g. single mothers, black youth, gay or lesbian, etc.). Being open in membership does not mean that the group is inclusive. But if it is exclusive, it must be able to clarify who it represents (its criteria for membership), and to be open to all those who meet these criteria. The group should also be able to develop some means to be accountable to those whom it claims to represent. This accountability ensures that the group does not become a small gathering of elites whose own sense of power is improved, but at the expense of a larger number of persons.

7. **The group is internally democratic**
    The group should not be authoritarian in its internal decision-making style. Authoritarianism is distinguished by:

    - unilateral decision making
    - censoring opposition within the group
    - controlling information
    - excluding others from leadership positions
    - favouring hierarchical forms of organisation, not because they may be more efficient for certain tasks, but because they allow a few persons to control the whole group

Adapted from Labonte (1998).

■ Marginalisation and indigenous people

Indigenous communities are a marginalised group to whom Simpson and Yinger's interpretation of a 'feeling of belonging or not belonging' has particular relevance. An example of indigenous communities living as a marginalised group within society is the Aboriginal and Torres Strait Islander people living in Australia. Aboriginal communities are often a collection of families, language groups or clans who can be in competition over limited resources and who may have been traditionally geographically isolated. The term 'community' was applied to the formation of the settlements or 'Aboriginal reserves' by bureaucratic intellectuals and those in authority because it provided a convenient label for the assimilation of a heterogeneous group of people (Scrimgeour, 1997). Inevitably, these 'artificial' communities led to conflict, family feuds and violence fuelled by the frustration of a lack of opportunities, low income and access to alcohol.

Goodman et al. (1998) argue that a sense of community can be strengthened through a connection with or an understanding of the history of the community. This is made up of events, people and experiences involving previous economic, political and socio-cultural contexts. Knowledge of the historical context of the community can help identify potential barriers to community empowerment such as experiences of conflict or feelings of helplessness. Goodman et al. (1998) argue that communities with access to information about their history, verbal or written, have a better chance of affecting change, than those that do not have access.

Story telling is an important part of Aboriginal culture and is the way communities pass down information about their history to put into context the reasons for their present day learned helplessness and internalised powerlessness. Psychological powerlessness, for example, the distress experienced with the unfairness of a lack of power and human rights is internalised as aspects of a sense of 'badness' or 'failure' and contributes to low self-esteem. The members of the marginalised group do not recognise that their circumstances are the result of wider structural reasons such as a weak government policy leading to a high level of unemployment, racism and social isolation.

Whilst not homogeneous, Aboriginal groups do largely share the same needs and interests especially in regard to public health. Whilst traditionally living a nomadic and remote, rural lifestyle, Aboriginal people mostly live in urban areas where they form a minority group. Aboriginal people experience a public health status well below the Australian average, for example, indicators of child survival rates, birth weight and the growth and nutrition of babies. Aboriginal infant and child health is significantly poorer than that of non-indigenous infants and children (Australian Bureau of Statistics, 2005). Much of the poor physical health of Aboriginal people has been related to their poor psychological health resulting from cultural disintegration, dispossession of their lands, unemployment, poverty and the feeling of not belonging to the wider society (marginalisation) in which they live (O'Connor and Parker, 1995). For example, in the 2001 Census, for example, 48% of Aboriginal people aged 15 years and over were reported to be unemployed in Australia (Australian Bureau of Statistics, 2001).

I next present a case study that describes how Practitioners worked with community-based organisations to strengthen the capacity of Aboriginal leadership to enable them to take more control of local health service delivery (Laverack, Hill, Akenson and Corrie, 2009). To protect the privacy of the members of the community the names of individuals and the identity of the location have not been used in the case studies.

■ A case study of helping Aboriginal community-based organisations to take more control of health service delivery in Australia

☐ Introduction

The importance of Aboriginal community control in service delivery to improve health outcomes has been recognised in both State and Federal Government policy for some time (Aboriginal and Torres Straight Islander Health Policy (1994; National Strategic Framework for Aboriginal and Torres Strait Islander Health, 2003). Underpinning this health reform process is the need to build community capacity for Indigenous people to take control of and be responsible for their own health. Community capacity building describes a process that increases the assets and attributes that a community is able to draw upon in order to improve their lives and health. In practice what this means is facilitating an increase in community groups' abilities to define, evaluate, analyse and act on concerns of importance to their members.

The approach was used as a starting point in the process of capacity building in the recently established Health Action Teams (HATs), the local health advisory groups in some remote Aboriginal communities. The HATs aim to have representation that considers the cultural make up of each community and draws from as many families and Clan Groups as possible. They also strive to involve representation from existing community-based organisations including the council, primary health care centre, men's and women's groups, justice groups, aged care, homelands, Community Development Employment Program (CDEP) and the women's centre. Members must be recognised by the community as local community members. The purpose was to build the capacity of the HATs in three remote Indigenous communities: community K; community C and; community L in far north Queensland. All three communities are characterised by remoteness with access only by flights or long drives, and all experience several months of the year where they are cut off by road due to the wet season. Each community has a range of other outreach services including medical, child health, drug and alcohol, community liaison development, health promotion, allied health and mental health.

☐ Building the capacity of the community-based organisations

To build the capacity of the community-based organisations, the HATs, an established approach was used (Laverack 2006) employing eight domains (see Table 6.1). The domains serve as a framework for building HAT capacity and represent those aspects that allow its members to better organise and mobilise themselves towards gaining greater control of local health services. Each domain was discussed with the HATs prior to implementation of the approach to further adapt their interpretation. The approach was implemented as a workshop. Each workshop was attended by the HAT members and held over a one to two day period in their

Table 6.1 Capacity 'domains' for Aboriginal communities in Australia

Domain	Interpretation
HAT participation	Participation is basic to building capacity. Only by participating can individual members better define, analyse and act on issues of concern to the broader community that they represent.
Local leadership	Participation and leadership are closely connected. Leadership requires a strong participant base just as participation requires the direction and structure of strong HAT leadership. Both play an important role in the development of the community.
Problem assessment capacities	Capacity building presumes that the identification of problems, solutions to the problems and actions to resolve the problems are carried out by the HAT. This process assists them to develop a sense of self-determination and the skills necessary for greater community capacity.
Organisational structures	Organisational structures include committees such as the HAT and the Council. These represent the ways in which people come together in order to address their concerns and problems. The existence of and the level at which these function is crucial to building capacity.
Resource mobilisation	The ability of the HAT to mobilise resources both from within and the ability to negotiate resources from beyond itself is an important factor to achieve successes in its efforts towards capacity building.
Links to others	Links with people and organisations, including partnerships, coalitions and alliances between the HAT and others, can assist the community in more effectively addressing its issues.
Ability to 'ask why'	The ability of the HAT to critically assess the social, political, economic and other causes of inequalities is a crucial stage towards developing appropriate personal and social change strategies for capacity and empowerment.
Health Services Management	Control should extend to decisions over planning, implementation, evaluation, finances and administration of the health services. The first step is to have clearly defined roles and responsibilities of all the stakeholders with outside services acting to support community capacity.

community. The purpose of the workshop was to firstly measure HAT capacity and then to formulate a strategic plan to address identified weaknesses. To do this, the HAT members used the 'domains approach' that is discussed in detail in Chapter 7. The measurement is in itself insufficient to build the capacity of the HAT who must also have the ability to transform this information into action. This is achieved through strategic planning for positive changes in each of the domains using three simple steps: a discussion on how to improve the present situation; the development of a strategy to improve upon the present situation; and the identification of any necessary resources. The measurement and strategic plan for each domain were then summarised in a table which formed the basis for further discussions, planning, and action. The table and spider-web configuration were both documented and given to all HAT members for future follow-up and reassessments of HAT capacity in collaboration with the outside services.

☐ The public health outcomes

Community K has a population of approximately 1110 people of which 85% are Indigenous and is located 740 km or approximately nine hours drive from the regional centre of Cairns. Community K HAT is comprised of ten members, four males and six females. Feedback from the HAT indicated that they found this a useful tool to determine their strengths and weaknesses and were able to develop a realistic plan for improving their capacity. In general, capacity was quite low as the HAT was in the early stages of establishment. Participation was ranked the highest as the members reported active involvement in monthly meetings. The need to obtain support from leaders outside the HAT and being recognised by the wider community as the peak local health advisory group was identified as a key strategy to build capacity. The strategy developed included a range of marketing and promotional activities and the development of a Memorandum of Understanding between the HAT and the Shire Council. Training was another strategy identified by the HAT to develop skills in specific areas including resource mobilisation and (local) health problem assessment.

    Community C is located eight hours drive from the regional centre of Cairns. The community has a population of approximately 300 people in the dry season which increases as people come in from Outstations or Homelands during the wet season. Indigenous people make up over 80% of the local population composed of members of several language groups from the surrounding region. The non-indigenous population runs the local business enterprises and essential services with only a few indigenous people being employed locally. Community C HAT is a voluntary membership and comprised of six members, five women and one man. The measurement of capacity by the HAT team shows that there were existing strengths in participation, organisational structures and leadership. The HAT felt that participation in decision making by its members had been maintained, that this was promoted by the organisational structure of the group and that they had established mechanisms to share information. The HAT leadership was functioning well internally but did not have established links with other community leaders. In general, capacity was quite low, the HAT was in the early stages of development and had not established itself as a key community-based organisation. This latter issue was identified by the HAT as an important next step to build its capacity. The HAT and the Council were to draft and agree upon a formal Memorandum Of Understanding in regard to the roles and responsibilities of the HAT for the health reform of Aboriginal services. This was to be supported by each member taking the responsibility to visit an area of the community to inform householders about their role. The HAT was to also write a letter of introduction requesting a meeting with the Regional Aboriginal Corporation, Chamber of Commerce, Justice Group and other key organisations in the community. Another key strategy towards building HAT capacity was identified as the need for specific skills training on marketing and submission writing. The training would be organised by an outside service provider and delivered as a workshop in the community.

Community L is a remote Aboriginal Community on the east coast of Cape York and is about 850 km north of Cairns by road. During the wet season, creeks and rivers flood and close the road into town. Sea and air are the only access at this time which can extend from December until June. The community has a population of approximately 650 people of which 61% are Indigenous. The measurement of capacity by the HAT team showed a similar pattern of capacity as demonstrated in communities C and K. Community L HAT had strengths in participation, organisational structures and leadership but did not have a developed capacity in 'asking why', external linkages, health services management, resource mobilisation and problem assessment. This pattern of high and low capacity rating is typical in newly formed community-based organisations and the next step was to prepare a strategy to address a few of the weaker domains within a feasible timeframe.

The strategy included the following activities to build their capacity:

- Problem assessment, resource mobilisation and local leadership: Undergo specific training in participatory health needs assessment skills, submission writing and marketing and leadership skills to be organised by an outside service provider within three months;
- Organisational structures: Organise a community BBQ to raise awareness of the role and responsibility of the HAT. HAT to raise funds by submitting a proposal to an appropriate funder within three months;
- Links to others: Prepare a letter to be sent to the Council to request a meeting to clarify the roles and responsibilities of the HAT.

There were a number of similarities in the measurement of capacity between the three HATs. Firstly, each HAT identified strengths in participation and leadership and a need to improve external linkages, resource mobilisation and health problem assessment capacities. Each community rated their capacity for health service management and the ability to 'ask why' as very low. The overall capacity in each HAT was at about the same level because they had been established for about the same length of time. Building capacity is a process that strengthens participation, organisational structures and local leadership so that it is meaningful to carry out a problem assessment, to mobilise resources and to establish external linkages. At a later stage their capacity will have developed to further enable the HATs to engage with health services management and to take action on the underlying causes of community poverty and powerlessness ('asking why').

Each HAT recognised the importance for strategic planning in this process. This offered them with the means to link the measurement of capacity to tangible actions through their participation and planning. Each plan was to be followed by the HAT, supported by the outside service providers and a review of the strategic plans carried out. Each HAT also reported that the 'spider web' was an appropriate means of visual representation in an Aboriginal context to show the strengths and weaknesses in capacity. It helped to promote the free flow of information and allowed HAT members and outside services to visualise, better articulate and to share their ideas on the building of capacity towards health leadership.

As the only local advisory group on health in some Aboriginal communities there is an enormous amount of interest in the Health Action Team from both within the community and from visiting services. But the need for communities and supporting organisations to have realistic expectations of these newly formed groups is paramount. It is important that the HAT sets boundaries based on their measured capacity and scope of practice otherwise they run the real risk of failing in their attempts towards health reform.

HAT members are often faced with a range of competing priorities and are already balancing responsibilities including working full time and holding other key positions within the community. It is therefore important to have a clear plan for capacity building towards which each HAT member can commit themselves to make it work.

An important implication is how assistance is provided by the outside services to facilitate the transformation of information gained from the measurement, by the HAT, into the actions necessary to build their capacity. The documented strategic plan and the visual representation for capacity provided the focus around which the community and the outside services could begin to develop a 'partnership of cooperation'. This was defined by the level of support requested by the HAT to implement activities, based on the strategy it had developed, to directly strengthen its own capacity.

Capacity building concerns the development of skills and abilities that will enable others to take decisions and actions for themselves and therefore directly assists communities toward becoming empowered 'increased control over events that determine their lives (and health)' (Werner, 1988, p. 1). This is achieved by the development of strategies to support each of the domains where a need has been identified by the community. In turn this strengthens the social aspects of empowerment, for example, the existence of functional leadership, supported by established organisational structures with the participation of all its members who have demonstrated the ability to mobilise resources, would indicate a more cohesive community, which has begun to develop strong social support elements (Laverack, 2001). The process of empowerment strengthens the cohesiveness of the community and builds the competencies and skills of its members.

As discussed in Chapter 2, power in its simplest form is about control over decisions and choices, both at the individual and collective levels. In an Aboriginal context, this is a complex issue. The nomadic 'hunter-gatherer' culture of Aboriginal people was until recently the key to survival in a harsh environment. People were conditioned to be opportunistic and to take whatever was available at that time rather than having to make a rational decision about longer-term control, for example, over resources. The unwillingness to accept responsibility for personal and collective decisions is just one factor (others include 'humbug' or the obligation to share resources with relatives, a different 'world view' and low self-esteem) why empowerment must be seen as a long-term goal in Aboriginal communities (Cresswell, 2004).

■ Marginalisation and migration

Migration, either in terms of internal migration where no national boundaries are crossed, or international migration where people move to another place across national boundaries, occurs for a variety of reasons. For example, people may leave their home countries to look for better economic opportunities, because of oppressive political circumstances, to be with family, for education or because they are forced to move. Migration is not always intended to be permanent and many people may wish to return to their home country at some stage in the future. A significant factor in the evolution of how migration patterns have developed has been the advancement of the methods of travel (MacPherson and Gushulak, 2004).

Migrant communities can become socially and economically marginalised and Simpson and Yinger's (1965) interpretation of a 'feeling of belonging or not belonging', discussed earlier, has resonance for many migrants. Examples of migrants living as a marginalised group within society include ethnic minority groups such as Chinese and Turkish, religious groups such as Jewish and Muslim and illegal or seasonal workers. When living in a new country many migrants are faced with restricted legal rights, a poor understanding of the local language, culture and system, different spiritual beliefs and a low income. This can lead to feelings of marginalisation and alienation and as a consequence they can be placed in a more vulnerable position of poor physical and mental health. This is a situation that is compounded by the migrants having a limited understanding of how to access health care services.

I next present a case study that describes how Practitioners can work with recent Chinese migrants, in New Zealand, to improve health outcomes by preventing injuries in the home and by promoting health care and rehabilitation services.

■ A case study of helping Chinese migrants to take more control of their health by preventing injury from accidents in New Zealand

☐ Introduction

It is estimated that 9.1% of New Zealand's current population is 'Asian' and this proportion is projected to grow to almost 15% by 2020. In urban areas, for example in wider Auckland, it is estimated that 34% of the population will be 'Asian' by 2016. In particular, the number of new Chinese migrants continues to grow, for example, the People's Republic of China moved from the fourth most common birthplace in 2001 to the second most common in 2006 (Statistics New Zealand, 2007).

Adopting a new lifestyle in New Zealand can result in accidents and injuries and the most common forms of reported accidents among Asian people included accidents in the home and motor vehicle traffic injuries. Yet Asian migrants have little understanding of their entitlements to accident insurance cover, the healthcare system and rehabilitation services (ACC, 2006). Injury is a leading cause of premature death and disability in New Zealand where the Accident Compensation Corporation (ACC) offers and organises help to anyone in the event of injury. The support covers provisions of rehabilitation services and is mandated to cover injury related costs irrespective of the nature of the injuries and the place of occurrence. ACC deals with 1.4 million injury claims each year and the annual economic cost of injury is estimated to be $NZ6–7 billion. However, in 2006 only 4.6% of the 9.1% of Asians in New Zealand claimed for accident entitlements, well below the national average (ACC, 2006).

One Study (Tse, Laverack, Nayar and Foroughian, 2008) found four common themes specifically among recent Chinese migrants in Auckland in preventing injuries.

Theme 1: Resettlement and relocation issues
Recent Chinese migrants had different experiences and lifestyles 'back home'. Lack of familiarity with the New Zealand lifestyle and limited knowledge as to how to cater for different circumstances created a tendency for accidents and injuries to occur.

Theme 2: Lack of communication
Some Chinese migrants were confused about the function and services provided and attributed this to a lack of communication between the agencies and the community and the lack of such a service in their home country. Prior to sustaining an injury, most migrants knew about a rehabilitation service by name, however at the time of injury, they were not confident about accessing services. Language and a lack of resources, especially those translated into Chinese, were identified as barriers to engaging with the Chinese community in communication activities.

Theme 3: Deployment of Chinese media

Chinese migrants suggested a variety of channels through which the community could be better informed about available services and there was an emphasis on utilising Chinese media, Chinese newspapers, radio stations, websites and workshops.

Theme 4: Community readiness and building community capacity

Joining one or more community organisations is an ordinary practice for Chinese migrants, particularly new migrants, in which they hold a great deal of trust and confidence. Reasons identified in the study for using Chinese Community-Based Organisations (CCBOs) included socialising, networking, information gathering, and preserving many unique aspects of their culture. To engage with migrants it is therefore important that Practitioners build the capacity of the available CCBOs.

The themes identify some of the difficulties that Chinese migrants face when both preventing and accessing assistance for injuries. Chinese migrants are settling in New Zealand with little knowledge about the local health/injury rehabilitation services, compounded by communication and other barriers. In order to effectively engage Chinese migrants in public health interventions their voices have to be heard and their capacity has to be developed towards gaining more power. Practitioners can play an important role in building community empowerment to give migrants the knowledge, skills and competencies that they require to address their concerns, including injury prevention and rehabilitation.

☐ Assisting migrant Chinese to gain power

As discussed in Chapter 5 the 'domains' to build community empowerment focuses on nine areas of influence on the process of community empowerment:

1. Community participation;
2. Problem assessment capacities;
3. Local leadership;
4. Organisational structures;
5. Resource mobilisation;
6. Links to other organisations and people;
7. Ability to 'ask why' (critical awareness);
8. Community control over programme management; and
9. An equitable relationship with the Practitioner.

A description of each domain is provided in Table 5.2. These domains can also be used as a framework to build community empowerment in Chinese migrant communities. What follows is a description of the types of activities involved in strengthening each domain in a public health programme engaging with Chinese migrants.

☐   *Community participation*

A major challenge for many Practitioners is to develop and maintain the trust of migrant communities. This is a long-term process of dialogue and commitment. An important part of trust building is the continued delivery of service standards in a partnership that is seen to be equitable, fair and open. The practice challenge to build relationships within the migrant community is to encourage broader participation in group activities. Within the spatial dimension of 'the migrant community', multiple other 'communities of interest' exist and individuals may belong to several at the same time. Interest groups exist as a legitimate means by which migrants can participate in a more formal way to achieve their goals and address mutual concerns, for example, through the Chinese New Settlers Services Trust. There is also a variety of other CCBOs such as Chinese Student's Association, social clubs and groups for well-being and exercise that are supported by the broader Auckland regional Migrant Services. This is a 'one stop centre' to provide information, consultation and referral services for all migrants to assist with their relocation to a new country.

The role of the Practitioner is to continue to listen to the community and to respond to their needs. This will include the provision of information to support activities for capacity building using a mix of strategies and appropriate channels of communication. Tse, Laverack, Nayar and Foroughian (2008) found that an appropriate communication strategy for Chinese people included messages and materials in English, Mandarin and Cantonese distributed through a combination of the following channels: Chinese newspapers; Chinese TV (World TV [paid TV]); Chinese Radio stations; Public meetings/networking meetings; Chinese festivals; Chinese health promoters; Chinese health days; English language classes; Citizens Advice Bureau and Printed materials such as Leaflets and posters.

☐   *Problem assessment capacities*

The migrant community should be helped in the identification of their problems, solutions and actions. The success of a programme depends to a great extent on the commitment and involvement of the intended beneficiaries. People are much more likely to be committed if they have a sense of ownership in regard to the problems being addressed. Programmes that do not address community problems and that do not involve the community in the process of problem assessment usually do not achieve their purpose. There are a number of different tools that can be used to help communities to identify their problems, including a questionnaire or focus groups discussions, in regard to injury prevention. A meeting is held with different CCBOs typically beginning with a brief introduction to the purpose followed by an introduction of the participants. The meeting is a facilitated group discussion to focus on a particular issue such as accidents in the home and on other issues that may be introduced such as compensation procedures. The meeting can be supported by a video tape that can be used in CCBOs followed by a facilitated dialogue, for example, on the prevention of domestic accidents. The meeting can be used to plan for actions, identify resources, identify potential partners and for people to openly express their views. To encourage participation it is worthwhile advertising the meeting in advance using the Chinese media.

☐ *Local leadership*

Even in 'communities of interest' participation often means representation as not every member can be actively involved. Practitioners need to carefully consider if the representatives of a community are in fact supported by its members and that they are not simply acting out of self-interest. In these circumstances, a position of power-over can be gained by a dominant minority who then dictate the community needs which are based on their own concerns and not those of the majority. The Chinese migrant community in Auckland is comprised of a number of different socio-cultural groups including mainland Chinese, Hong Kong Chinese, Taiwanese, English, Mandarin and Cantonese speakers, youth and the elderly. Within an empowering approach the Practitioner does not have a role to direct the community how it should identify its representatives. The community must decide who should and who should not be their representatives. The Practitioner can help by ensuring all representatives have an equal opportunity to express their opinions and abide to the criteria for selecting community groups in Box 6.1.

At the beginning of the programme the leadership may be guided by a Practitioner who has regular consultations with migrant representatives. The local leaders of the Chinese New Settlers Services Trust, for example, are involved in the planning and administration of programmes and can receive training and instruction in management skills to build their capacity. The aims and objectives of the programme include the problems identified by the community. This would determine the roles and responsibilities that form the relationship between the migrant community and the Practitioners. The design is agreed as part of a framework for the implementation and evaluation of the programme.

☐ *Organisational structures*

It is important that an existing organisation(s) are involved in implementing the programme, in this case by a number of CCBOs with assistance from the Practitioner. To enable migrants to increase control of, and improve health through the management and prevention of injuries the programme can offer assistance to strengthen the organisational structures of the CCBOs. This would include the characteristics of successful interest groups identified by Jones and Laverack (2003):

1. Had a membership of elected representatives;
2. The majority of its members met on a regular basis;
3. Had an agreed membership structure (chairperson, secretary, core members, etc.);
4. All members actively participated in the meetings;
5. The group met with a Practitioner to discuss issues on a regular basis;
6. Kept records of previous meetings;
7. Kept financial accounts;

8. Were able to identify and resolve conflicts quickly; and
9. Were able to identify the 'problems' of and the resources available to the 'interest group'.

☐ *Resource mobilisation*

Migrant communities often have access to limited internal funds but can be rich in other resources such as human resources, connectedness, cultural identity and individual energy. In New Zealand, migrant communities are entitled to health care and rehabilitation services and to compensation for injury. The role of the Practitioner is to inform the migrants of the available services, their individual rights and to provide them with the necessary skills to access the available services, for example, the ability to complete an accident claim form, This information would include:

• Full services offered by the appropriate accident compensation agency, for example, How it operates, Who qualifies and under what situations, What and how much is covered, How and when one should make the claim.
• Where to access language support when using the appropriate accident compensation agency.
• Information regarding contact details of the registered Chinese therapists with the appropriate accident compensation agency and details of the private and/or public clinics/hospitals, which are covered by the appropriate accident compensation agency.
• Injury prevention measures for slips, falls, DIY injuries and domestic accidents such as scalding and cuts.
• Self-care, first aid and appropriate referral (Tse, Laverack, Nayar and Foroughian, 2008).

☐ *Links to other organisations and people*

Community links to other organisations and people, including the Practitioner, implies an equal partnership based on mutual respect, trust and a sharing of information and experiences. Community links with other people and organisations also include coalitions and alliances. The role of the Practitioner is to help the CCBOs, to develop partnerships with others who share their needs and concerns. Partnerships build the ability of the community to develop relationships with different groups or organisations based on recognition of overlapping or mutual interests, and inter-personal and inter-organisational respect. They also build the ability to network, collaborate, co-operate and to develop relationships that promote a heightened inter-dependency amongst its members. Working in partnership will lead toward greater political and social influence of individuals and groups through an expanded membership and resource base, for example, this might involve the development of pressure groups to advocate for better legislation of injury prevention (Laverack, 2007).

It is the role of the Practitioner to assist the migrants to engage with others to build different types of partnerships, for example, in Chinese communities it would be appropriate to develop both coalitions and alliances. Community-based coalitions can be defined as '...a group of individuals representing diverse organisations, factions, or constituencies within the community who agree to work together to achieve a common goal' (Butterfoss et al., 1996, p.66). Unlike partnerships, coalitions represent a diversity of views on a common issue and member groups have to learn to set aside differences and to deal with internal conflicts. The outputs of links with other organisations and individuals may include proposals, recruitment of new members and the generation of resources resulting in improvements for the majority of the people in the community.

Alliances can be described as a process that involves co-operation and collaboration to create a partnership between organisations and individuals to enable people to increase control over the factors that influence their lives. It is a collaboration that through the collective efforts of its members' attempts to bring about broader social, political and environmental change to positively influence their needs (Jones, Sidell and Douglas, 2002), for example, a change in legislation or policy regarding Chinese people. An example of an alliance in the Chinese community might include the collaboration between for example, the Chinese New Settlers Services Trust and the Citizen Advice Bureau.

☐ *Ability to 'ask why' (critical awareness)*

Some Chinese migrants have come from a political context in which organisational structures at all levels are inherently top-down and function within a rigid and controlled bureaucratic apparatus. Civil society is a relatively new concept and some migrants are not use to the egalitarian conditions in New Zealand that are meant to facilitate critical awareness. 'Asking why' is distinct from the domain of problem assessment capacities in that it encourages CCBOs to think beyond their immediate concerns and to take a stronger position on broader issues. Therefore rather than using a top-down didactic approach the Practitioner can help the community members to work together in small groups to analyse why some people were more prone to accidents and injuries than others and what local and national actions might remedy their particular circumstances. Through these group discussions migrants can also gradually become more critically aware of the broader issues of their powerlessness in a process of discussion, reflection and action. The most suitable approach is to use a 'facilitated dialogue' between the community and the Practitioner to allow the knowledge and priorities of both to decide an appropriate direction for the programme.

☐ *Community control over the programme management and an equitable relationship with the Practitioner*

A programme in which the Practitioner directs assistance at the community can serve to reinforce a sense of subordination. This creates the practical dilemma of finding ways to assist community empowerment, in a programme context, without reinforcing dependency. The first challenge is to identify the communities' own sources of power (resources, decision-making authority, technical skills, local knowledge etc). Rather than begin from the perspective that migrants are, in general terms, 'relatively' economically and politically powerless. The Practitioner looks for, and works from, areas in peoples' lives in which they are 'relatively' powerful. For example, migrants may hold a great deal of authority in one aspect of their life, such as being a community leader, but possess very little authority in other aspects, for example in the workplace they may have only a low-paying menial job with little responsibility. Local leaders can be an important factor in enabling others to take control of the influences on their lives and health and to help manage programmes once they have the skills and competencies. Transferring responsibility for management is a long-term and ongoing process but over time, and as additional resources and skills are obtained, the community can take on more control. This includes activities such as management, fund-raising and liaison with other organisations and people. This can be facilitated by having a systematic approach that aims to give more responsibility to migrants for their management and involvement in the programme. The second challenge is to assist migrants to organise and mobilise themselves collectively through strengthening each of the 'empowerment domains'. The third challenge is to support the creation of an adequate resource base for community action and to do this the Practitioner can act as a link between external resources, such as government grants, and the community (Laverack, 2007).

Next, in Chapter 7, I discuss an approach to specifically measure empowerment through each of the nine 'domains' (discussed in Chapter 5) and a 'spider web' configuration to visually represent and interpret this information. I illustrate this approach with a case study of empowering rural communities to take control of local resources in Thailand.

Chapter 7

The measurement and visual representation of community empowerment

■ Collecting and analysing qualitative information

Public health programme design and evaluation is often based on the use of participatory techniques, qualitative and quantitative methods. In empowerment approaches qualitative techniques, such as one to one and focus group interviews, are especially useful to draw upon the knowledge and experiences of clients. I therefore begin this Chapter on the measurement of community empowerment with a discussion about collecting and analysing qualitative information in both a western and cross cultural context.

In qualitative interviewing, the aim is to discover the interviewee's own framework of meanings and to avoid imposing the interviewer's structures and assumptions as far as possible. The interviewer needs to remain open to the possibility that the concepts and variables that emerge may be very different from those that might have been predicted at the outset. The interviewer needs to be sensitive to the language and concepts used by the interviewee and check that they have understood the meanings of the respondent. The flexibility of the interviewing technique will allow a change in the pace and direction and this can be used by the interviewer to avoid any misunderstandings during the inquiry (Britten, 1995).

☐ Qualitative interviewing

Two main interview types can be used; unstructured and semi-structured. Unstructured interviews may cover only one or two issues and whilst semi-structured interviews are also conducted on a loose structure consisting of open-ended questions that define the area to be explored, the interviewer may diverge in order to pursue an idea in more detail and depth.

The less structured the interview, the less the questions are determined and standardised in advance of the interview. However, most interviews will have a list of core questions that define the areas to be covered (Britten, 1995). Questions should be open ended, neutral, sensitive and clear to the interviewee, usually starting with questions that the interviewee can easily answer and then proceeding to more difficult and sensitive topics.

☐   Starting the inquiry to collect qualitative information

The initial part of the inquiry uses unstructured interviews with key informants to identify the main themes of power and empowerment in the specific cultural context. Unstructured one-to-one interviews are used to discover the interviewee's own framework of meanings. This type of interview dispenses with formal schedules and ordering of questions and relies on the social interaction between the interviewer and the informant to elicit information (Minichiello et al., 1990). The unstructured interview takes on the appearance of a normal everyday conversation. However, it is always a controlled conversation, which is geared to the interviewer's interests. The element of control is minimal but present in order to keep the informant 'relating to experiences and attitudes that are relevant to the problem' (Burgess, 1982, p. 107). More than one unstructured interview can be used so that further questions could be based on what previous interviews had said and these should consist mostly of clarification and probing for more depth and detail. It is important to carry out as many unstructured interviews as are necessary to be sure that all the main headings for power and empowerment have been identified. The interviewees can be different but the interviews are to be based on the same themes of power and empowerment. They ought to begin with the interviewer asking 'This interview is about power in your cultural context. Can you tell me about your experiences, what you think this means and how it works in your communities?' The interviews can be held at the interviewees' places of work, homes or in a neutral setting, at a predetermined and convenient time. The interviews must be recorded either manually or by using a tape-recorder and normally ought to last between 30 and 90 minutes.

☐   Gaining in-depth information

The findings of the unstructured interviews provide the main headings for the next part of the inquiry, semi-structured group interviews. The questions do not have a fixed order or wording, but act as a guide to the interviewer who uses them in small groups consisting of stakeholders of similar characteristics. The purpose of the interviews is to provide more depth and comprehension to the main headings and to provide anecdotal information to highlight the findings. Questions are developed in regard to the key terms to determine who has power and how the different forms of power interrelate. The sample selection for the interviews is undertaken to ensure a representative range of age and socio-economic background of the interviewees in the community.

Group interviews are a quick and convenient way to simultaneously collect data from several people. This means that instead of the interviewer asking each person to respond to a question in turn, there is some interaction and people are encouraged to talk, ask questions, exchange anecdotes and to comment on each others' experiences. Some of the potential advantages are that the technique does not discriminate against people who cannot read or write and encourages participation and discussion especially from those who might normally feel that they have nothing to say. However, the articulation of group norms may silence individual voices of dissent and it is these contradictions that the interviewer may want to gain access to as a part of the findings. The presence of other interviewees may also compromise the confidentiality of the session, however, groups are not always inhibiting and may actively facilitate the discussion of taboo topics. Participants may provide mutual support in expressing feelings that are common to the group (Kitzinger, 1995).

The success of the group interviews depends on both the skill of the facilitator and the discussion environment. Sessions should be relaxed, in a comfortable and familiar setting, refreshments may be available and the seating should be arranged in a circle or sequence acceptable to the participants. The facilitator should be able to 'take a back seat' but also be able to use debate to continue the conversation beyond the stage where it might have otherwise ended. The facilitator should be able to use disagreement to encourage participants to elucidate their point of view and to clarify why they think as they do. Basically, the facilitator should be sensitive to the group and to its particular dynamics (Minichiello et al., 1990; Kitzinger, 1995).

☐ Keeping a record of the inquiry

A number of different notes can be used by the interviewer to help compile a record of events, for example, a simple notebook can be used to keep detailed records of events, conversations, activities and descriptions. The type of notes can be distinguished as either mental jottings and full notes. Mental notes are made of discussions or observations after the event, jotted notes are quick, short hand notes to remind the interviewer of events. Full field notes are the running notes made throughout the day during or after the observational period and are both descriptive and analytical. The descriptive notes portray the context in which the observations and discussions took place. The analytical notes try to make sense of what has been observed and may be made after the observation when the interviewer has more time to reflect and clarify his or her impressions (Glesne and Peshkin, 1992).

☐ Analysing the qualitative information

The aim of the analysis of the qualitative information is to look for areas of common ground and differences between the respondents of the interviews rather than provide a number of separate accounts. The recommended procedure for analysis uses a cut and paste technique which is quick, simple and cost effective for small amounts of qualitative data. The information, which is available in the form of field notes and transcribed interviews, goes through a process of disaggregation and reaggregation using the following steps:

1. The process of disaggregation begins when photocopies are made of the original field notes. The copies are used to identify a classification system for

the major categories of discussion. The categories are identified in the text by using coloured marker pens to highlight their presence in the text. The recorded text is thoroughly reread and all the marked relevant phrases, sentences or exchanges of recorded conversation are checked.

2. Once the colour coding is complete the marked text is cut up and sorted into files that have been marked one for each category. The categories will form the headings of the discussion of the findings.

3. The process of reaggregation happens by rereading each category file to analyse the content in its new context alongside information of a similar nature. New insights and confirmations begin to emerge and the structure of the findings and discussion begin to form.

■ Collecting and analysing qualitative information in a cross-cultural context

Public health programmes can involve different cultural groups in which the Practitioner is of a different ethnicity and is seen as an outside agent by the clients. Before collecting qualitative information in a cross cultural context there are issues which need to be taken into account, for example, the unfamiliarity with a specific cultural context makes it more difficult for a Practitioner to reflect the reality of the situation. This means that important information might be lost during the interpretation across cultures (Cuthbert, 1985). The most significant difficulties faced by Practitioners have been their inability to speak the local language, holding a different belief and value system, poor communication and different styles of interaction, social relationships, attitudes towards time, infra-structure and political sensitivities (Merryfield, 1985). It is recognised that knowledge of the local language, whilst important, is not essential, and that building a rapport with potential clients is more a function of time spent on site and of interpersonal skills than it is of cultural identity and linguistics (Ginsberg, 1988).

In practice it may not be possible to have a facilitated group discussion due to the language and cultural differences between the Practitioner and clients. In this case, a facilitated design can be used that takes the cultural context into account. This requires a facilitator to be appointed to work with the Practitioner, one who is familiar with the cultural context. Facilitation introduces higher levels of control, the ability to focus on specific goals within a limited time period and is not merely translation or interpretation. Apart from 'process' skills of accurate interpreting and 'back translation' to the Practitioner during the course of the meeting, the ways in which facilitators work in the group setting as well as their role, style, background and appearance is crucial in shaping interactions.

Figure 7.1 provides a typology of roles that a facilitator can play during any cross-cultural group meeting. Based on the levels of facilitator direction (leading and control techniques) and rapport (trust-building and distance reducing techniques), four general types of role can be delineated: empathy; engagement; railroading and disengagement (Laverack and Brown, 2003). Empathy involves the facilitator being able to achieve insightful understandings based on taking the point of view of the other. This is most likely when rapport (an equivalence of meaning construction between parties) is high and facilitator direction is low. Engagement also requires high rapport together with greater levels of facilitator direction, for example, where the facilitator encourages a particular direction for discussion. Low rapport results in role types that should be avoided. When rapport is lost or not gained, higher direction can force discussion to areas of lesser interest to the participants and is a kind of railroading. Low rapport combined with low levels of direction can leave the facilitator as a disengaged 'outsider' whose observations may lack validity. In practice, movement occurs between role types as the group meeting progresses whereas the arrows in Figure 7.1 represent an ideal facilitation model with an interplay of engagement and empathy that characterise the duration of the group meeting. High rapport is maintained and direction levels lowered and raised optimally according to the flow of the group interaction.

The requirement for good facilitation is crucial to many aspects of qualitative research. Cross cultural facilitators are able to speak the local language, understand local customs and more easily explain complex concepts without the need for translation and this will help to expedite the meeting. Stewart and Shamdasani (1990) point out that personal bias by facilitators in focus groups, who tend to direct the discussion and reinforce certain points of view, is a phenomenon common to Westernised cultures.

Laverack and Brown (2003) also found that in a non-westernised context facilitators tended to: lead the discussion and took a directive, rather than a

Figure 7.1 Facilitator role types

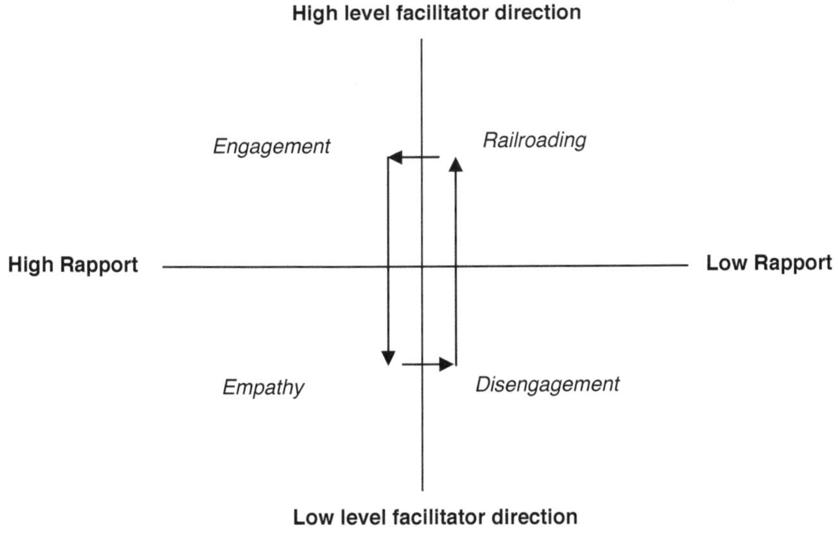

High level facilitator direction

Engagement   Railroading

High Rapport ———————————————— **Low Rapport**

Empathy   Disengagement

Low level facilitator direction

Adapted from Laverack and Brown, 2003, p. 4.

participatory approach (railroading); encourage discussion but did not try to involve all the participants (loss of rapport); dominate and directed group interaction and it was observed that they did not allow the focus of discussion to move towards its members as the workshop progressed (too directive); and left the room and the participants were very able to continue each exercise but control of the discussion resumed with the facilitators upon their return (too directive).

Skilful facilitation is an issue common to qualitative approaches and the question; 'how to ensure proper facilitation?' constantly needs to be addressed. This includes the maintenance of a good standard of facilitation skills in order to aim consistently for a successful balance between direction and rapport. Possessing the necessary skills and experience does not guarantee against facilitator bias but proper training may reduce unintentional influences.

While high rapport is always the goal of skilful facilitation, in a cross-cultural context this may have to be achieved through roles embodying lower levels of rapport and differing levels of engagement. The purpose of this approach is to better position the facilitators to achieve an empathetic understanding of the participants. Cross-cultural contexts can provide essentially novel or unique issues and problems. The facilitators may have to be prepared to be more and less directive and engaged when collecting qualitative information, adapting their approach to the specific requirements of the participants. This can be described as an 'inward' and 'outward' movement by the facilitators towards a terrain of empathy conveying a similar pattern to those noted in qualitative and participant observatory research (Glesne and Peshkin, 1992). A key feature, and therefore a key skill of facilitation, in these circumstances is the ability of the facilitator to correctly identify the moments of transition and apply an empowering language (discussed in Chapter 4).

In general, there are two other categories when working in a cross-cultural context that can be improved: the use of appropriate technologies; and the engagement of suitable personnel. Appropriate technologies for collecting cross-cultural information have been identified as a more naturalistic approach; the use of qualitative methods such as case studies and interviews which use the strong narrative and oral traditions of different cultures (Cuthbert, 1985; Russon, 1995). The approach should use both qualitative and quantitative information to cross-check the findings. The technologies should also be flexible in terms of time and attitudes, be participatory and use culturally sensitive instruments for data collection (Cuthbert, 1985; Merryfield, 1985).

The skills and personal qualities required of the people collecting the cross-cultural information have been identified as: tolerance for ambiguity; patience; adaptiveness; capacity for tacit learning; and courtesy (Seefeldt, 1985). A number of authors have suggested that a team comprising both foreign personnel and facilitators from the host community, preferably someone working closely with the public health programme, provides the most suitable approach (Chow et al., 1996; Cuthbert, 1985; Westwood and Brous, 1993). When it is not possible to work in a team, or if a local person is not available, then adequate training about the cultural context should be provided to anyone not from the specific cultural context (Russon, 1995). It is also important for the outside agent to have a prior understanding of the fluid social dynamics and complex balance of relationships that occur between programme stakeholders in a cross cultural context. Activities that may have little or no relevance to the Practitioner, such as the seating arrangements in a meeting, may have profound implications for the clients. This understanding can be improved through cross cultural awareness training and the provision of better communication skills (Cass et al., 2002).

The measurement of community empowerment

Of the different levels of empowerment it has been the psychological element which has received the most attention in terms of measurement (Rissel et al., 1996; Zimmerman and Rappaport, 1988; Zimmerman and Zahniser, 1991). Other authors have used predetermined indicators of outcome as a part of external assessments of empowerment in a programme context (Barr, 1995; IRED, 1997; Labonte, 1994). These indicators cover a range of social, political and economic factors relating to the level of control that a community has over the influences on their lives. The measurement of empowerment has also traditionally used qualitative information to provide 'thick' descriptive accounts, based on the experiences of the participants, which produce a large quantity of data such as transcribed interviews. This type of data is difficult and time consuming for Practitioners to analyse and to interpret. The trade off is between the use of timely but not so in-depth generic approaches such as standardised checklists with the more locally appropriate information procured from participatory 'tools' which are potentially time consuming. The aim of an empowering approach to measurement is to strengthen the design, to provide all stakeholders with a mutual understanding of the programme and to make Practitioners more sensitive to differences in meaning such as the cultural context, as discussed in Chapter 2.

Few authors discuss the development of a practical approach for the measurement of community empowerment that is based on sound research and thorough field testing. However, I next discuss an approach that is robust and for which there is substantial evidence of its potential as a participatory tool to build and measure community empowerment.

The 'domains approach'

The 'domains approach' gives a precise way in which to strengthen and measure concepts such as community capacity and community empowerment. Specifically the approach uses nine 'domains' which are the areas of influence on the process of community empowerment. Details of the identification and interpretation of the 'domains' of community empowerment are provided elsewhere in Laverack (2001) and in Chapter 5. A summary of each domain are provided in Table 5.2. What follows is a brief description of the methodology for the 'domains approach', including a visual representation of the measurement, followed by a case study example of its implementation in Thailand.

The 'domains approach' is used with community members or their representatives and is usually facilitated by a Practitioner. The participants are first provided with five qualitative statements for each of the nine empowerment domains, written on a separate sheet of paper. The five statements for each domain are provided in Table 7.1 and represent a range of empowering situations but each statement can also be rewritten by the participants to reflect the actual situation in their community. Taking one domain at a time, the participants are asked to select the statement that most closely describes the present situation in their community. The statements are not numbered or marked in any way and each is read out loud to encourage group discussion. The selection of a statement by the participants is then based on their own experiences and knowledge (Laverack, 2003).

Next, it is important that the participants record the reasons justifying the measurement for each selected domain. This assists other people who make subsequent measurements and who need to take the previous record into account. It also provides some defensible or empirically observable criteria for the selection. This overcomes one of the weaknesses in the use of qualitative statements, that of reliability over time or across different participants making the assessment (Uphoff, 1991). The justification needs to include verifiable examples of the actual experiences of the participants taken from their community to illustrate in more detail the reasoning behind the selection of the statement.

The sum of the measurement is a set of nine qualitative statements, one for each domain, which represent the strengths and weaknesses of empowerment in the community at that particular time. The five statements for each domain are pre-ranked or pre-rated from one (least empowering) to five (most empowering). The ratings are not shared with the participants during the measurement to avoid the introduction of bias. Laverack (1999) found that the use of pre-quantified rating scales unacceptably influenced the behaviour and actions of the participants. The participants progressively ranked themselves higher for each domain compared with a methodology that did not allow them to have any prior knowledge of the rating scale. The use of the rating scales led to the introduction of subject bias such that the participants did not make an independent assessment but instead provided consistently high ratings to match the expectations of their members. Each selected qualitative statement is rated by the facilitator, following the measurement, to give it a quantitative value that can then be used to plot the data. For example, for the domain 'Local leadership' (see Table 7.1) if the participants choose the statement 'Leaders exist for all community organisations. Some organisations not functioning under their leaders', this domain will be plotted with a rating of 2. In practice any numerical value can be given to the five statements depending on the type of graphical plot that the facilitator wishes to make. The measurement, analysis and interpretation of this information should be shared with everyone, from policy makers 'down' to the community members. The information may also have to be compared over a specific time frame and between the different components

Table 7.1 The ranking for each generic empowerment statement

Domain	1.	2.	3.	4.	5.
Community participation	Not all community members and groups are participating in community activities and meetings such as women, youth, men.	Community members are attending meetings but not involved in discussion and helping.	Community members involved in discussions but not in decisions on planning and implementation. Limited to activities such as voluntary labour and financial donations.	Community members involved in decisions on planning and implementation. Mechanism exists to share information between members.	Participation in decision making has been maintained. Community members involved in activities outside the community.
Problem assessment capacities	No problem assessment undertaken by the community.	Community lacks skills and awareness to carry out an assessment.	Community has skills. Problems and priorities identified by the community. Did not involve participation of all sectors of the community.	Community identified problems, solutions and actions. Assessment used to strengthen community planning.	Community continues to identify and is the owner of problems, solutions and actions.
Local leadership	Some community organisations without a leader.	Leaders exist for all community organisations. Some organisations not functioning under their leaders.	Community organisations functioning under leaders. Some Organisations do not have the support of leaders outside the community.	Leaders are taking initiative with support from their organisations. Leaders require skills training.	Leaders taking full initiative. Organisations in full support. Leaders work with outside groups to gain resources.

Table 7.1 The ranking for each generic empowerment statement – *continued*

Domain	1.	2.	3.	4.	5.
Organisational structures	Community has no organisational structures such as committees.	Organisations have been established by the community but are not active.	More than one organisation which are active. Organisations have mechanism to allow its members to provide meaningful participation.	Many organisations have established links with each other within the community.	Organisations actively involved in and outside the community. Community committed to its own and to other organisations.
Resource mobilisation	Resources are not being mobilised by the community.	Only rich and influential people mobilise resources raised by community. Community members are made to give resources.	Community has increasingly supplied resources, but no collective decision about distribution. Resources raised have had limited benefits.	Resources raised also used for activities outside the community. Discussion by community on distribution but not fairly distributed.	Considerable resources raised and community decide on distribution. Resources fairly distributed.
Links to others	None.	Community has informal links with other organisations and people. Does not have a well defined purpose.	Community has agreed links but not involved in community activities and development.	Links inter-dependant, defined and involved in community development. Based on mutual respect.	Links generating resources, finances and recruiting new members. Decisions resulting in improvements for the community.

Table 7.1 The ranking for each generic empowerment statement – *continued*

Domain	1.	2.	3.	4.	5.
Ability to 'ask why'	No group discussions held to ask why about community issues.	Small group discussions are being held to ask 'why' about community issues and to challenge received wisdom.	Groups held to listen about community issues. These have the ability to reflect on assumptions underlying their ideas and actions. Are able to challenge received wisdom.	Dialogue between community groups to identify solutions, self-test and analyse. Some experience of testing solutions.	Community groups have ability to self analyse and improve its efforts overtime. This is leading toward collective change.
Programme management	By agent.	By agent in discussion with community.	By community supervised by agent. Decision-making mechanisms mutually agreed Roles and responsibility clearly defined. Community has not received skills training in programme management.	By community in planning, policy and evaluation with limited assistance from agent. Developing sense of community ownership.	Community self manage independent of agent. Management is accountable.
Relationship with outside agent	Agents in control of policy, policy, finances, resources and evaluation of the programme.	Agents in control but discuss with community. No decision making by community. Agent acting on behalf of agency to produce outputs.	Agents and community make joint decisions. Role of agent mutually agreed.	Community makes decisions with support from agents. Agent facilitates change by training and support.	Agents facilitate change at request of community who makes the decisions. Agent acts on behalf of the community to build capacity.

Adapted from Laverack, 1999.

of a programme. For this purpose, visual representations of the measurement of community empowerment can be an appropriate way to interpret and share the information.

■ The visual representation of the measurement

Several authors have used visual representations to compare changes in the factors that can influence the process of community empowerment and other community-based approaches. For example, John Roughan (1986), a community development Practitioner, devised a wheel configuration and used rating scales to measure three areas: personal growth; material growth and social growth for village development in the Solomon Islands. The rating scale had ten points that radiated outwards like the spokes of a wheel for each indicator of the three growth areas. Each scale was plotted following an evaluation by the village members to provide a visual representation of growth and development. The approach used a total of 18 complex, interrelated indicators such as equity and solidarity to evaluate village development.

Rifkin et al. (1988) in Nepal and later Bjaras et al. (1991) in Sweden, were the first commentators on the use of the 'spider-web' configuration for the visual representation of community participation. Their approach identifies five factors: leadership; needs evaluation; management; organisation and resource mobilisation, and uses a similar simple rating scale. The approach was not carried out as a self-evaluation by the community and did not promote strategic planning. However, these early experiences of measurement have provided the basis for subsequent attempts with visual representation. For example, Marion Gibbon (1999), a community development Practitioner, in her measurement of community capacity in Nepal utilised a set of eight domains, similar to those independently developed by Laverack (1999), and a set of indicators with a rank assigned from 1 (low) to 4 (high).

Rankings of measurement have been graphically plotted using a configuration similar to the spider-web approach used by Rifkin et al. (1988). Different stakeholders in the same programme use the visual representation to make comparisons of each domain during the life of the programme. The spider-web configuration has been used with some success for visual representation and has also been urged by several of the community empowerment models (Bopp et al., 1999; Hawe et al., 2000; Laverack, 1999). The spider-web can be an especially useful tool when using a 'domains approach', as discussed earlier, because the assessment of each domain can be visually communicated and shared by all stakeholders. The spider-web also provides a quick picture of the strengths and weaknesses within a community (defined by the nine domains) and between communities in the same programme.

Next, I provide a case study (Laverack and Thangphet, 2007) of how one agency in Thailand has used the domains approach to build and measure community capacity towards the self-management of local ecotourism projects. The purpose was to give the communities more control (power) over their environment and the employment opportunities it offered to lead to better health and well-being of their members. Some approaches have an explicit purpose to empower people by bringing about social and political change and this is embodied in their sense of action and political activism (Laverack, 2007, p. 29). Other approaches begin with a focus on individual, group or community participation, action and capacity building. Community empowerment and community capacity overlap closely as forms of social organisation and mobilisation that seek to address the inequalities in peoples lives (Laverack, 2007, p. 19). Capacity building is often the means by which the outcome of community empowerment can be achieved through systematically building knowledge, skills and competencies at a local level. Building community capacity is not isolated to a single outcome. The skills and competencies developed can be transferable across social, political and economic issues at the community level. At some point the community recognises that there is the need for an agenda of activities in order for people to gain access to political influence and resources at a broader level. This then moves the community from engaging in a strategy of capacity building to one of empowerment.

■ A case study of empowering rural communities to take control of local resources in Thailand

☐ Introduction

Economic and social development programmes have increasingly placed an emphasis on sustainability. In pursuing this direction, the concept of community capacity building has become of particular importance in identifying priorities and opportunities for development (Victurine, 2000). The International Ecotourism Society defines ecotourism as 'responsible travel to natural areas which conserves the environment and improves the welfare of the local people. A walk through the rainforest, for example, is not ecotourism unless that particular walk somehow benefits that environment and the people who live there or a rafting trip is only ecotourism if it raises awareness and funds to help protect the watershed' (Untamed Path, 2007, p. 1). Ecotourism is therefore also closely linked to conservation and sustainable environmental development.

Community-Based Ecotourism has been seen by the Thai Government as a means to raise the income of rural people as well as conserving their culture and the environment. Both Government and Non-Government Organisations have been involved in training villagers to work in tourism and typically tours are organised so that visitors can experience the local culture. There has also been a history of some villagers acting as guides, porters and accommodation providers in the form of home-stays (Anucha, 2001). However, the rapid development of tourism has tended to overlook the ability of communities to maintain these enterprises and whether they fully address the interests of their members, of the tourism industry and of environmental conservation (Adis, 1996). In reality few stakeholders, including communities, in the Northern provinces have had much experience in managing ecotourism as they have used relatively new forms of tourism such as cultural immersion. In the South of the country the Thai economy is heavily reliant on conventional forms of tourism and there is therefore a real need to build capacity in the Northern provinces to address both community needs and to contribute towards the national agenda on ecotourism.

☐ The cultural context

The approach to build community capacity was implemented in two Northern Thai ecotourism enterprises in Chiang Mai province, Northern Thailand: Ban Tam-Nong Bia and Ban Mae kampong, with the support of the Nagao Natural Environment Foundation.

☐ Ban Tam-Nong Bia community

Ban Tam-Nong Bia is located in Sri Dongyen sub-district, Chaiprakhan district, Chiang Mai province. It is 120 km north of Chiang Mai city along Chiang Mai-Fang road, 2 km from the main road along a small asphalt access road. The topographical feature of the village is a narrow valley surrounded by mountain ranges. The village covers an area of five square kilometers and has an approximate population of 623 persons comprised of 170 households. About 70% of the villagers are engaged in seasonally paid work in the agricultural sector, for example, in lychee and longan fruit orchards. The average household income is about US$25 per month (Thangphet, 2006, p. 22). The community was able to estimate that 5,000–6,000 tourists visited their area annually mostly to visit the Wat Tamtabtao, a famous Buddhist temple. However, the community had gained little benefit from this source of tourism as the usual pattern was a one day visit where tourists returned to their hotel in another area. An ecotourism project was started in 2003 to attract tourists to the village, for example, cultural performances, and the community wanted to build its capacity to better manage this opportunity.

☐ Ban Mae Kampong community

Ban Mae Kampong is in Huai Kaew sub-district, Mae On district, Chiang Mai province. It is an upland village, located 50 km northeast of Chiang Mai city along the Mae On-Huai Kaew Road. The village got its name from its physical characteristic of having several streams passing through the community. The early settlers migrated from Doi Saket district, the nearby district in Chiang Mai province, to search for land for forest-tea orchard cultivation. The topographical feature of the area is a hilly terrain at an elevation of 1,000 m above sea level. The village is divided into six clusters, covering an area of approximately 6 square kilometers.

The village has a population of approximately 418 persons and 130 households. About 97% of villagers are engaged in fermented tea production, locally called 'miang.' However, in recent years, the villagers have turned to growing coffee by planting it in the forest-tea gardens. This crop diversification occurred in response to the decline of fermented tea production and has now resulted in an average household income of about US$90 per month (Thangphet, 2006, p. 40).

☐ Experiences of building community capacity

Prior to implementation the interpretation of each domain was discussed and adapted in consultation with the stakeholders to ensure that they were relevant within the context of Thailand and the Project. The approach was implemented as a series of participatory workshops in each community to measure community capacity and to formulate a strategic plan to address identified weaknesses. Approximately 30 key stakeholders from each community participated in the workshops. The nine domains were used to measure community capacity towards the management of ecotourism enterprises. The domains served as a framework for community capacity and represented those aspects that allowed individuals and groups to better organise and mobilise themselves towards gaining greater control of locally managed ecotourism.

The workshops were organised at the community center or in the temple and the participants included the village headman, community ecotourism committee, community ecotourism members, occupation group leaders, and local villagers. The facilitator guided the participants through the approach, discussed earlier, to make a measurement and then to develop a strategy to improve each of the domains. The following is a brief account of follow-up interviews that were carried out in each community two months after the first workshop to gain an insight into the experiences of building community capacity.

☐ The Ban Tam-Nong Bia community

The approach had enabled the community to identify those domains that needed urgent action for improving the management capability for ecotourism. This process was greatly facilitated by the use of the spider-web (Figure 7.2) which allowed all community members (literate and non-literate) to understand the strengths and weaknesses in their capacity.

The spider-web in Figure 7.2 shows a distribution of high and low ratings of the nine domains, indicating a range of strengths and weaknesses in capacity in Ban Tam-Nong Bia community. Leadership was ranked the highest. This person was a village headman and he had initiated the development of the cultural immersion for tourists as a form of ecotourism. Participation was ranked as being one of the lowest domains by the community. Many villagers still had to find work outside their community and this had resulted in them not being involved in the decision

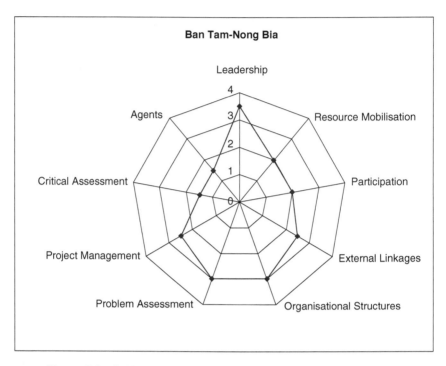

Figure 7.2 Spider web configuration for Ban Tam-Nong Bia community

making process concerning community ecotourism. The leadership role had been significant in carrying the local enterprise forward but the villagers felt that better participation of the community was essential to promote sustainability. They therefore decided to develop a strategic plan to promote participation as a priority over other domains that had also received a low ranking. This was to be achieved through training and linkages with external organisations for future collaboration on ecotourism activities.

The ecotourism leader of Ban Mae Kampong community served as a trainer to share the experiences of their success in ecotourism. These included the benefits of the hospitality management, ecotourism management, and the process used to mobilise community participation. In addition, this exchange helped to strengthen the informal network between the two community ecotourism enterprises. Ban Tam-Nong Bia has a variety of ecotourism resources but there were few local guides available to provide information and tours for the tourists. An external organisation provided training for local guides and helped to collect community information about its history, resources and local customs. Ban Tam-Nong Bia decided to develop its own ecotourism website to promote tourism and to establish links with other ecotourism organisations. The skills necessary to do this were also provided through links with an external organisation based in Thailand.

☐   The Ban Mae Kampong community

The approach had engaged the villagers in a process of problem solving and an analysis of the information taken from the capacity assessment to strengthen community management. This process led to a consensus for how to improve ecotourism in their community. The leader had organised a further workshop to discuss the issue of community participation and how the ecotourism enterprise would benefit everyone in the community. Discussion was facilitated by referring to the spider-web for community capacity (Figure 7.3) in which several domains had received a high ranking. This is an indication that the overall capacity in Ban Mae Kampong was high at the time of the assessment. Leadership was ranked the highest score because the present leader played an essential role in initiating and sustaining the community ecotourism. He was responsible for all ecotourism activities and a dominant figure in conflict mediation between project and non-project beneficiaries. Despite the strong leadership, the domains for an equitable relationship with outside agents, participation, and critical assessment received a lower ranking. These domains were identified as being weaker because the present leader did not have the skills to adequately direct the future development of community ecotourism. The community developed strategies to improve upon this situation including ecotourism training, the use of home-stays, hospitality management skills and the design of a website for the community activities.

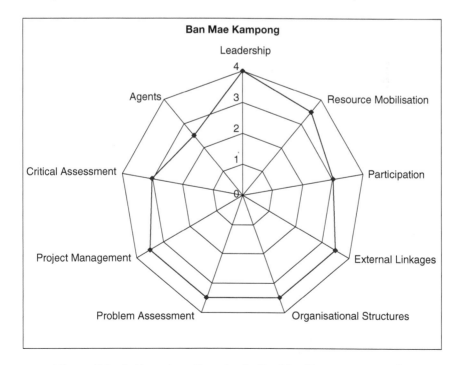

Figure 7.3   Spider web configuration for Ban Mae Kampong community

Existing government laws and regulations were seen by the community as an obstacle to their effective management of ecotourism. The community had no legal right to manage the public resources in its area, such as public land and forest resources, for ecotourism. Without a legal recognition, the community was unable to use public resources for community ecotourism purposes. In response, the community decided to establish a link with the local government authority to help legitimise community regulations and to defend its customary rights to use public resources. Through this link the local government granted permission to the community to use the public resources and helped to enforce the community regulations on any people who violated the agreement. To get this approval the community therefore had to organise and mobilise itself to lobby the local authority, represent itself through strong leadership and to raise common interest within the community to show its strengths through collective participation. This experience had increased the sense of self-determination in the community.

In Ban Mae Kampong, the community ecotourism had been developed for conserving the community resources, particularly forest resources, and generated employment for local people to police the illegal forestry activities. Due to its rapid success, more attention had been given to income generation and the community felt that the principles of community ecotourism were essential for the long-term sustainability. A training workshop was organised by an 'expert' on ecotourism and conservation, partially sponsored by community funds, and this helped to provide a clearer understanding of their role in ecotourism toward natural resource conservation. The workshop provided examples of other local successes in this area and the local villagers were encouraged to share their experiences with other communities.

The community also felt it was important to promote the home-stay approach for tourists to experience rural Thai culture. The ecotourism leader explained to community members about the minimum requirements of the accommodation, catering and how to meet the needs of the tourists. Linked to this was training in hospitality management. This one-day training was organised at the community center and gave villagers the confidence to cater for home-stay visitors. To facilitate better access to the tourism market the community also developed a website for community ecotourism. The website provided the background of the community, a history of its community ecotourism development, community ecotourism resources and activities. The experiences of building community capacity in Ban Mae Kampong, illustrated that for community-based action to thrive there is also the need for a supportive and enabling environment. This can be facilitated by Government policy and regulations that promote locally managed ecotourism, for example, local control over publicly owned resources. Alternatively, governments can provide support through access to funding sources that promote community development.

The use of a means of visual representation of the measurement of community capacity, in this case study used the form of a spider-web to promote discussion in what is traditionally an oral and visually orientated culture. For example, in Ban Tam-Nong Bia community the spider-web configuration allowed both literate and non-literate villagers to visualise, articulate and share their ideas on the building of community capacity. This was especially useful when trying to engage the community members to participate in the ecotourism enterprise. In Ban Tam-Nong Bia community the leadership role had been significant in carrying the enterprise forward but participation by community members was poor. Broader participation would be essential for the future development and sustainability of locally managed ecotourism. The spider-web provided an easily understandable method for the leaders to communicate this issue to the community members and to mobilise their support for the enterprise. The leader used the spider-web of community capacity to visually explain the strengths and weaknesses of the community and this promoted more active participation by the villagers.

Next, in Chapter 8, I bring together the central themes of the book, power and empowerment, and draw conclusions about the present and for the future of public health programming.

Chapter 8

The future of public health programming

In this book I have argued that power and empowerment are central to public health programming. I have also argued that Practitioners are faced with constraints when trying to use a more empowering approach in their work. In this the final Chapter, I discuss where we are presently and what the future of public health programming will have to look like in order to be both more empowering and more successful in achieving its goals.

■ Why we are where we are

Public health programming is predominately top-down, pre-packaged, has a biomedical focus and is professionally driven in which the Practitioner exerts control through implementation, management and evaluation (Laverack, 2004, 2007). Top-down programming is based on scientific evidence such as epidemiological studies and addresses population issues such as the increase in obesity, cancers, dangerous consumptions such as smoking and violence and injury (Wanless, 2003). Practitioners have found it difficult to use empowerment approaches in their everyday work in top-down programming (Loss and Wise, 2007). Empowerment or bottom-up approaches assist the community to identify its own problems and to communicate these to the top structures. The role of the Practitioner is to enable their clients to identify solutions and actions to address their problems by providing technical support, resources and by building capacity. Problem assessment, as I discuss in Chapter 3, is often an important first step for Practitioners to engage with communities and to begin the facilitation of individual and collective empowerment. Bottom-up agendas address local problems such as community safety, anti-social behaviour and an untidy environment (Liew, 2007) as well as public transport, housing standards and social exclusion (Laverack, 2008).

The two agendas (top-down and bottom-up) do not therefore always share the same goals and this can create a 'top-down versus bottom-up tension'. National (top-down) public health agendas are typically centred on improving health through, for example, promoting healthy lifestyles, physical activity and modification of the diet. The lifestyle agenda has proved attractive to many political leaders because it promised easily quantifiable and achievable results within a short time frame, it dealt with high prevalence health problems such as obesity, was simple (Gangolli, Duggal and Shukla, 2005) and offered powerful future cost-savings in health care services for people suffering from chronic diseases such as diabetes and heart disease (Bernier, 2007). It also shifted the focus away from awkward political issues concerning the underlying health determinants rooted in poverty and inequality (Labonte and Laverack, 2008). Communities on the other hand are more concerned with their immediate problems such as high unemployment or reducing crime in their neighbourhood and have not been motivated by a top-down agenda and the programme activities that it offers.

Over the years top-down public health programming has had only a modest success in achieving its goals, for example, a review of 155 programmes in the USA found that almost all had been unsuccessful (Freudenburg, 1997). There is further evidence that the modest success of top-down programming has only been with higher socio-economic groups. In Australia over the period 1998–2004 there was a 9% decrease in smoking in the lowest quintile compared to a 35% decrease in the highest quintile (Baum, 2007, p. 91). In Canada over the period 2000–2005 a top-down programme to increase physical activity in urban and rural communities found that 30% people had become more active whilst 14% had become less active. Significantly, the change in physical activity had occurred in the higher socio-economic groups with little or no effect on low socio-economic, adolescents, ethnic minorities or indigenous people (SRHA, 2005).

Top-down programming has relied heavily on strategies of the behavioural sciences and has largely employed health education modelling to raise awareness levels and to bring about individual behaviour change. Health education messaging has in some cases remained unchanged for many decades, for example, in regard to daily physical exercise and nutrition. Health education has also used clear and simple messages that have been informed by the latest scientific evidence. Despite this health education approaches have been found to be ineffective except with the educated and economically advantaged in society (Nutbeam, 2000) who have the skills and economic base to respond to improve or protect their health. As a consequence, top-down programming may have had no effect in closing the gap between the healthy wealthy and low socio-economic groups. It may even, at least temporarily, have led to an increase in inequalities in health (Baum, 2007; Nutbeam, 2000). In certain circumstances this may have been made worse by public sector cuts that reduce health prevention and promotion services to the poor or by weakened safeguards on harmful goods such as access to and advertising on junk food. The ability of the wealthy to afford the many health services and products offered by the private sector, estimated to be worth $200 billion in the USA, has also been largely inaccessible to the poor (Kickbusch, 2002).

The modest success achieved through top-down public health programming has not been because of the issues it chooses to address or the messages it chooses to communicate. It has been because of the way in which public health programmes have been delivered. Top-down programming has relied heavily on strategies that have not engaged with poor and marginalised people. Low participation in and motivation for top-down programming has hindered its progress to achieve the primary goal of closing the gap in health status between different social and economic groups in society.

As public health programming moves into the twenty-first century there is a further dimension to take into consideration; Globalisation. At its simplest, globalisation describes a constellation of processes by which nations, businesses and people are becoming more connected and interdependent through increased economic integration and communication exchange, cultural diffusion and travel (Diamond, 1997). Disease has inevitably followed its path as trade and travel have long been vectors for epidemics. Crucially, for over 20 years public health has recognised the centrality, if not primacy, of the physical environment as a prerequisite to health. Virtually all environmental markers show deterioration in our life support. Climate change is undoubtedly the most urgent health issue and its linkage to global market integration is straightforward: Moving goods around the world consumes fossil fuel and exhausts greenhouse gases (Labonte and Laverack, 2008). Public health programming must take into consideration how it will contribute to the global health agenda by also addressing, for example, the issues of climate change, fossil fuel consumption, trade and employment, pandemics and biological security (Wanless, 2003).

■ What public health programming will have to look like in the future

In the future all public health programming will have to better accommodate the three health agendas discussed above (see Figure 8.1):

1. National agendas based on population studies and empirical scientific evidence to address, for example, the rise in obesity, cancers and dangerous consumptions;
2. Community agendas to address local problems such as community safety, anti-social behaviour, unemployment, public transport, housing standards and social exclusion;
3. Global agendas by addressing, for example, the issues of climate change, fossil fuel consumption, trade and employment, pandemics and national security (Laverack, 2008).

Simply put, this means in practice, for example, that a national agenda on reducing obesity through an increase in physical activity will also have to address local problems such as an unsafe environment in low socio-economic communities. In turn this will contribute to a global agenda by a reduction in fossil fuel consumption because more people are walking to the local shopping centre rather than using their motor vehicles for personal safety. There are examples that have been successful in combining both top-down and bottom-up elements in their design such as the 'like minds, like mine' national level project which aimed to counter stigma and discrimination associated with mental illness in New Zealand. This project evolved by using a combination of top-down mass media and community education, building community leadership and participation, developing an infrastructure that also had culturally specific approaches (MoH, NZ, 2003). But to

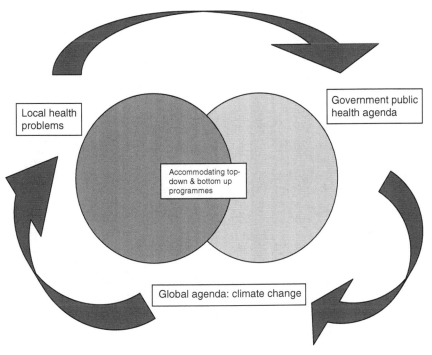

Figure 8.1 The future of public health programming

achieve the successful combination of all three agendas in the future public health programming with have to address how:

1. Engage communities to share their priorities;
2. Build community capacity;
3. Have mechanisms for flexible funding;
4. Evaluate and share information and ideas;
5. Be creative to expand on successful local initiatives (Laverack, 2008).

■ Engage communities to share their priorities

A major step to improving public health programming in the future will be to better accommodate top-down and bottom-up agendas. The key to this is for Practitioners to engage with communities during the planning process to identify their problems and then to incorporate these concerns within the design of the programme. Problem assessment strategies for communities and accommodating top-down and bottom-up agendas is discussed in Chapter 3. Engaging with people in a programme context is crucial but it is not straight-forward, for example, research in the UK has shown that of 80% of people who claimed to want to get involved in public services when further questioned only 25% were actually prepared to give up their time (Confederation of British Industry 2006).

Public health programmes in the future will only be successful if they can maintain a high level of participation and motivation of their clients. Box 8.1 provides an example of how one local council engaged with communities to improve the delivery of public services.

Engaging people to address local concerns can be facilitated by using innovative ways to build partnerships and alliances with other stakeholders. This is especially important when working with ethnic minorities, indigenous and low socio-economic groups who are sometimes marginalised within public health programmes. The engagement can often be based on a problem that has already been identified by the community, what I call a 'community wedge', to provide a point of mutual interest around which the programme can develop. Box 8.2 provides an example of engaging a community to take responsibility on some of the tough questions in regard to a local road maintenance project.

It is important to maintain a proper balance between professional and community inputs as sometimes conflict can occur over a lack of clarity about who has the decision-making authority (Anderson et al., 2006). But even when devolution includes both resources and authority, many Practitioners find it difficult to relinquish the control that they have over the design and implementation of a programme (Syme, 1997). Accepting the expertise offered by local people and sharing professional expertise so that the members can build their own empower-

---

Box 8.1 Improving the Delivery of Local Services in the UK

Slough Borough Council in the UK set up a citizen's jury to decide how to improve their 'street-scene' services in response to concerns primarily from local residents. This included road maintenance and street cleaning. This was a new initiative to create a partnership between the Council and local residents and other stakeholders. A new delivery strategy was devised to bring refuse collection and disposal, recycling, street cleaning, grounds and highways maintenance into a single partnership. At that time these contracts were split between different contractors. The Slough Borough council was given a mandate to increase Council Tax to improve the service, so long as the benefits could be guaranteed. A consultative board met every six months to help set service priorities, solve delivery problems and take forward campaigning and educational work. As a consequence local services improved rapidly and Slough is now one of the cleanest towns in the South of England. The 'Keep Slough green and tidy' campaign motivates the public to be actively engaged in the effort to increase recycling and decrease litter. The partnership has given local residents more of a 'voice' and has included them in the decision-making process to improve the environment in Slough (Confederation of British Industry, 2006).

Box 8.2 Improving Local Involvement in Road Maintenance in the UK

A private company was asked by the Oxfordshire County Council to develop a solution to increase the life of a major road in Oxford, UK including junctions, access and traffic calming. The work was planned to interfere as little as possible with local businesses and residents, by avoiding busy seasons and working when premises were closed. Road-user groups, local businesses and the police were involved from the design phase through regular public meetings. Residents were asked to choose from a series of options for the difficult decisions, such as when to work at busy junctions. The work itself was broken down into sections covering 200m of road and residents were told dates in advance and businesses were allowed to continue deliveries. The road maintenance was planned around the convenience of local residents and businesses who were also involved in making decisions on an ongoing basis. This was formalised as a 'neighbourhood charter' or a two-way partnership between communities and a service provider such as a construction contractor.

The partnership helped to ensure that the work started and finished on time by helping to identify problems in advance, and resulted in a higher level of local participation and client satisfaction. Other projects have employed a Watchman-in-Chief who engages with business, service users, parish councils, the Highways Agency and local representatives. Other watchmen identify issues across the area and feed back to the Watchman-in-Chief. The Watch-keeper role provides a non-bureaucratic, informal method through which the outside agency can keep in touch with a range of stakeholders when appropriate, enabling a feedback and communication. The information provided is realistic and accurate and always allows local residents to provide their opinions and, if necessary, to be involved with the decision-making processes (Confederation of British Industry, 2006).

ing capacities can be difficult for some Practitioners. The aim is to facilitate the sharing of power in a way that involves the provision of both services and resources, at the request of the community, in a culturally and socially acceptable manner. This is power-with, discussed in Chapter 2. Partnerships therefore offer a framework in which the relationship between the Practitioner and their clients can become more equal.

■ Build community capacity

Successful public health programming must have a clearly defined strategy of how it will build community capacity from planning, through implementation and management, to evaluation. Community capacity is achieved through systematically building knowledge, skills and competencies at a local level. Without this focus the community can become dependent on an outside agency to provide support and resources during the lifecycle of the programme without themselves taking greater control. Capacity building includes two key areas:

1. Firstly, the capacity of the community is strengthened so that members can better define, assess, analyse and act on health (or any other) concerns. This involves the development of specific skills which contribute to their overall capacity, and which are captured in the empowerment domains described in Chapters 5 and 7. These skills may be used later to sustain the programme outputs or to address a variety of other circumstances and therefore capacity building has a generic characteristic that is not limited to addressing only one issue.
2. Secondly, the capacity of the community to take more control of the programme is enhanced. This often involves skills development based on programme management such as financial control, report writing and participatory evaluation. These are skills that the community can use when it is involved in managing programmes.

Interest in community capacity building as a strategy for sustainable skills, resources and commitments in various public health programmes has developed because of the requirement to prolong programme gains (Gibbon et al., 2002). Community empowerment and community capacity overlap closely as forms of social organisation and mobilisation that seek to redress the inequalities in peoples' lives, often through programming (Laverack, 2007, p. 19). This process begins (as I discussed in Chapter 3) by building community capacity for problem assessment and using this information to design a programme that addresses both community priorities and public health (programme) priorities.

■ Mechanisms for flexible funding

Capacity building often involves the provision of resources to support local initiatives. To meet this demand the outside agent should be flexible in the type and timing of resources that they are prepared to provide to support the community. In a programme context resources are often designated to a specific budget category, for example, health education and screening services, which may not meet the resources requested for community initiatives, for example, refreshments for a meeting. These activities may be difficult to justify as strictly 'public health' but that nonetheless build the social dimension of communities through a sense of belonging, connectedness and personal relationships. Funding bodies must be able to think outside the 'health box' to be able to develop suitable prototypes for financial support, for example, for matching counterpart contributions, covering recurrent community costs, private sector involvement and models of 'users pay'

Box 8.3 Seed Funding Small Scale Initiatives

Joan Wharf Higgins et al. (2007) in British Columbia, Canada looked at 12 regional seed funded (short-term grants up to $4500 Canadian) initiatives for chronic disease prevention. They found that those initiatives with most capacity building had a better chance of success especially if resources could be found for the longer term as seed funding was too short to allow organic growth of the organisation. The conclusion was that ten out of the 11 initiatives continued beyond the funded period and that these types of partnerships between communities and government agencies can work towards achieving sustainability.

for a service or product delivery (Commonwealth of Australia, 2000). Actual examples of how health funding bodies have used resources to support locally-based initiatives include school and community gardens in Canada, the safer parks scheme in New Zealand (Gee, 2008), walking school buses in Australia, virtual communities in the USA and the green gyms and allotment junkies in the UK (CDC, 2006).

If the Practitioner does not have budgetary control then they still have a role of lobbying the funding body for programme delivery to use community empowerment/capacity-building approaches. However, funding agencies are often reluctant to take risks with resources for programme activities which they feel are unpredictable or that cannot be measured. One way of reducing the risk of a programme not achieving its goals is for the community to establish a joint venture, for example, between government, private and public interests (Anderson et al., 2006). Funding small scale initiatives can be a useful way to determine the validity of a programme design with a view to expand on successful community outcomes in such a partnership. Box 8.3 provides the findings of a study in Canada to determine the usefulness of funding small scale initiatives through seed funding.

■ Evaluate to share information and ideas

Although there is no real agreement about the overall purpose of evaluation in public health programmes it should address the concerns of all the stakeholders who require information about its impact, operation, progress and achievements. Funding agencies will want to see value for money, Practitioners will want to see improvements in health and communities will want to see their problems being resolved.

In top-down programming, evaluation can be used as an instrument of control through performance measurement of achieving targets by monitoring the operational elements of the implementation. The evaluation typically uses predetermined indicators, toward which the community members do not contribute, and is often implemented by an outside 'expert'. Bottom-up programming places the focus on participatory self-evaluation and away from conventional 'expert' driven approaches. This means a fundamental shift in the power relationship between the Practitioner and the beneficiaries of the programme, one where control over decisions about design and evaluation are more equitably distributed.

An evaluation that empowers ensures that it addresses local concerns and provides the information that people need to make better-informed decisions that go beyond the programme's own goals. Evaluation that empowers emphasises people being actively involved in the evaluation process. The evaluation itself then becomes an empowering experience by building the capacity of community members. Apart from evaluation of specific programme objectives there is the matter of tracking change in the complex concept of empowerment itself. Empowerment can be viewed as both a process and an outcome. By measuring empowerment as a process, it is possible to monitor the interaction between capacities, skills, and resources during the timeframe of a public health programme. (Labonte and Laverack, 2008). In the future public health programming will have to reach a compromise between top-down and bottom-up styles of evaluation. In Chapter 7 I discuss a participatory approach that can also quantify and visually represent the process of community empowerment. This approach uses elements of both top-down and bottom-up evaluation that can be understood by all stakeholders and has been used effectively to share information and ideas.

■ Be creative to expand on local initiatives

A key turning point in the empowerment of a community is when it stops focusing solely on its immediate needs and begins to address issues that have a broader concern. The process may begin with a local problem that has been identified by the community, for example, used syringes being left in a public park. Through the support offered by the programme this local problem develops into an understanding of the underlying causes of lack of control and a discussion about the broader determinants of their lives and health, for example, how the syringes are a symptom of anti-social behaviour by adolescents. Continued support by the programme leads to capacity building and an increase in knowledge and skills toward broader social and political action, for example, lobbying for better policing and an improved policy on cleaning and monitoring public parks. This action has the potential to develop further into community actions including other programmes that engage people to address local problems supported by public health agencies. However this will only happen if funding bodies are willing to be creative to scale-up or expand upon successful local initiatives and to allow bottom-up approaches to develop within top-down programming.

Scaling-up remains an important unresolved question. Would governments, taking an evidence-based approach to policy, be able to scale-up, in partnership with community-based organisations, to ensure benefits at a population level? Obviously this requires the right level of political commitment but scaling-up for empowerment and health across populations has been achieved for example in Bangladesh through partnerships such as the Bangladesh Rural Advancement Committee and the Grameen Bank. Women in Bangladeshi communities became more empowered through micro-financing with the help of the Grameen Bank. The loans were small and intended to give women more control over decisions regarding income generation and health. The success of the outcomes and loan repayments was attributed to the solidarity of small community organisations, social support and the financial advantage offered by the loan. By the beginning of 2005, the bank had loaned over USD4.7 billion, and by 2006 it had more than 2,100 branches in the country (Wheat, 1997; Papa et al., 2006).

Whilst there is no real agreement on the amount of increase that a programme has to obtain in order to reach a 'scale-up' it is usually considered to be the coverage of benefits to as many of the population within a specified area as possible, more quickly, more equitably and more lastingly (Core Group, 2005). The problem begins when pilot or demonstration projects are not planned to be scaled-up even when successful and are delivered as high cost and low participant activities. Scaling-up requires a planned process to be in place to expand on successful local initiatives once they have been 'field tested' through, for example, adding a creative initiative to an existing larger top-down programme (as discussed in Chapter 3 using parallel-tracking).

Programme experiences of scaling-up have shown that certain principles apply when expanding on creative local initiatives and these include:

- pilot test and evaluate a mature initiative to determine its successfulness and feasibility to go to scale;
- include all stakeholders (multi-sectoral) in the scale-up process from the beginning;
- scale-up to be inline with broader policy;
- promote human rights, equity and equality (Ayaonline.org, 2008).

Whether working with existing groups or new ones, in a partnership or directly engaging with the community, the roles and responsibilities of who facilitates the 'scaling-up' process must be clearly defined. Small scale projects are often successful because they are structured in such a way as to accommodate the power relationships at a local level. 'Going to scale' can result in these power dynamics becoming disrupted and roles at a local level not being acknowledged in a meaningful way. The impact, intentional or not, can have an effect on the 'scaling-up' process, for example, through a lack of participation, lower community contributions such as voluntary labour not being made or uncompleted activities such as building infrastructure (Earle et al., 2004). Expanding on successful local initiatives is important to gain greater and more equitable benefits but this process must be sensitive to the issue of power and empowerment, as discussed in this book, at both a local and broader level.

The spirit in which this book has been written is for Practitioners to consciously use the information provided to purposefully share power-with clients and not use it as a means to gain power-over them. The extent to which this happens will depend on how far Practitioners are willing to relinquish control in their everyday work and how honest Practitioners are prepared to be about their role in achieving an empowering practice. Given the constraints faced by many Practitioners this is a challenge. In this book, I explain how agencies, and the Practitioners that they employ, can use simple strategies to make their work more empowering in public health practice. The book offers a gradual way forward to develop public health rather than calling for a radical reorientation of practice. The way forward is more empowering for both Practitioners and their clients, wherever and with whoever they work. Essentially the challenge to build an empowering practice in the future lies with the public health profession and the Practitioners it employs. Together they will have to find creative ways, some of which are provided in this book, to motivate and enable others to share power.

References

Aboriginal and Torres Straight Islander Health Policy (1994) Queensland Health; Retrieved from www.health.qld.gov.au/indigenous_health/atsihp1994.pdf (6/2/2008)

Accident Compensation Corporation (ACC) (2006). Entitlement claims to ACC from July 2004–June 2005. Unpublished statistics for Asian ethnic groups.

Adis, I. (1996) Ecotourism. *TDRI Quarterly Review* 2: 10–15.

Adams, R. N. (1977) 'Power in human societies: a synthesis', in Fogelson, R. D. and Adams, R. N. (eds) *The Anthropology of Power: Ethnographic Studies from Asia, Oceania, and the New World*, pp. 387–410. New York: Academic Press.

Allmark, P. and Tod, A. (2006) 'How should public health professionals engage with lay epidemiology?', *Journal of Medical Ethics*, 32: 460–3.

Allsop, J., Jones, K. and Baggott, R. (2004) 'Health consumer groups in the UK: A new social movement', *Sociology of Health & Illness*, 26(6): 737–56.

Anderson, E., Shepard, M. and Salisbury, C. (2006) 'Taking off the suit': engaging the community in primary health care decision-making, *Health Expectations*, 9: 70–80.

Anucha, L. (2001) Changing Ecotourism to Community-Based Ecotourism in Thailand. Paper prepared for the Second Australian National Thai Studies. Melbourne: Royal Melbourne Institute of Technology.

Aggleton, P. (1991) *Health*. London: Routledge.

Appadurai, A. (2004) 'The capacity to aspire: Culture and the terms of recognition', in Rao, V. and Walton, M. (eds) *Culture and Public Action*, Chapter 3. California: Stanford University Press.

Asthana, S. (1994) 'Community participation in health and development', in Phillips, D. and Verhasselt, Y. (eds) *Health and Development*, pp. 182–96. London: Routledge.

Australian Bureau of Statistics and Australian Institute of Health and Welfare, *The Health and Welfare of Australia's Aboriginal and Torres Strait Islander Peoples, 2005*, ABS cat. no. 4704.0, Commonwealth of Australia, Canberra, 2005, p. 79.

Australian Bureau of Statistics, *Population Characteristics: Aboriginal and Torres Strait Islander Australians 2001, op.cit.*, p. 65.

Ayaonline.org (2008) 'Scaling-up'. Accessed on 30/4/2008. http://www.ayaonline.org/Strategies/PDFs/ScalingUp.pdf.

Baggott, R. (2000) *Public Health: Policy and Politics*. London: St. Martin's Press.

Barnes, M. (2002) 'User movements, community development and health promotion', in Adams, L., Amos, M. and Munro, J. *Promoting Health: Politics and Practice*. London: Sage Publications.

Barr, A. (1995) 'Empowering communities beyond fashionable rhetoric? Some reflections on Scottish experience', *Community Development Journal*, 30(2): 121–32.

Barrig, M. (1990) 'Women and development in Peru: old models, new actors', *Community Development Journal*, 25(4): 377–85.

Bassett, S. F. and Prapavessis, H. (2007) 'Home-based physical therapy intervention with adherence-enhancing strategies versus clinic based management for patients with ankle sprains', *Physical Therapy*, 87(9): 1132–43.

Baum, F. (1990) 'The new public health: force for change or reaction?', *Health Promotion International*, 5(2): 145–50.

Baum, F. (2007) 'Cracking the nut of health equity: top down and bottom up pressure for action on the social determinants of health', *IUHPE Promotion and Education*, 14(2): 90–5.

Bernier, N. (2007) 'Health promotion program resilience and policy trajectories: A comparison of three provinces', in M. O'Neill, et al. (eds) *Health Promotion in Canada: Critical Perspectives*. Toronto: Canadian Scholars' Press Inc.

127

Bjaras, G., Haglund, B. J. A. and Rifkin, S. (1991) 'A new approach to community participation evaluation', *Health Promotion International*, 6(3): 1999–2006.

Bloor, M. and McIntosh, J. (1990) 'Surveillance and concealment', in Cunningham-Burley, S. and McKeganey, N. P. (eds) *Readings in Medical Sociology*. New York: Tavistock/Routledge.

Bopp, M., Germann, K., Bopp, J., Littlejohns, L. B. and Smith, N. (1999) *Evaluating Community Capacity for Change*. Calgary: Four Worlds Development.

Boutilier, M. (1993) *The Effectiveness of Community Action in Health Promotion: A Research Perspective*. Toronto: University of Toronto, ParticiACTION. 3.

Bracht, N. and Tsouros, A. (1990) 'Principles and strategies of effective community participation', *Health Promotion International*, 5(3): 199–208.

Britten, N. (1995) 'Qualitative interviews in medical research', *British Medical Journal*, 311: 251–3.

Brown, P. and Zavestoski, S. (2004) 'Social movements in health: an introduction', *Sociology of Health & Illness*, 26(6): 679–94.

Brown, P., Zavestoski, S., McCormick, S., Mayer, B., Morello-Frosch, R. and Gasior, R. (2004) 'Embodied health movements: uncharted territory in social movement research', *Sociology of Health & Illness*, 26(1): 50–80.

Brunner, E. (1996) 'The social and biological basis of cardiovascular disease in office workers', in Blane, D., Brunner, E. and Wilkinson, R. (eds) *Health and Social Organisation: Towards a Health Policy for the 21st Century*. New York: Routledge.

Burgess, R. G. (1982) *Field Research: A Source Book and Field Manual*. London: Allen & Unwin.

Butterfoss, F. D., Goodman, R. M. and Wandersman, A. (1996) 'Community coalitions for prevention and health promotion: factors predicting satisfaction, participation and planning', *Health Education Quarterly*, 23(1): 65–79.

Cass, A., Lowell, A., Christie, M., Snelling, P. L., Flack, M., Marrnganyin, B. and Brown, I. (2002) 'Sharing the true stories: improving communication between Aboriginal patients and health care workers', *The Medical Journal of Australia*, 176(10): 466–70.

Centre for Disease Control and Prevention (CDC) (2006) 'Recommendations for future efforts in community health promotion. Regional expert panel on community health promotion'. Atlanta, USA.

Confederation of British Industry (CBI) (2006) Transforming Local Services. Confederation of British Industry Brief. London. July 2006.

Chow, J., Murry, S. and Angeli, C. (1996) International and multicultural teaming: a kaleidoscope of kolors. Annual conference of the American Evaluation Association. Atlanta: Indiana University.

Clegg, S. R. (1989) *Frameworks of Power*. London: Sage Publications.

Coleman, P. T. (2000) 'Power and conflict', in Deutsch, M. and Coleman, P. T. (2000) (eds) *The Handbook of Conflict Resolution. Theory and Practice*. San Francisco, CA.: Jossey-Bass Publishers.

Commonwealth of Australia (2000) Promoting practical sustainability. Canberra. AusAID.

CORE Group (2005) 'Scale' and 'Scaling-Up': A CORE Group Background Paper on 'Scaling-Up' Maternal, Newborn and Child Health Services. Washington DC: The World Bank. July 2005.

Cracknell, B. E. (1996) 'Evaluating development aid', *Evaluation*, 2(1): 23–33.

Cresswell, H. (2004) Personal email correspondence, 14/5/2004.

Cuthbert, M. (1985) 'Evaluation encounters in third world settings: a Caribbean perspective', in Patton, M. Q. (ed.) *Culture and Evaluation*. San Francisco, CA.: Jossey-Bass: 29–35.

Diamond, J. (1997) *Guns, Germs and Steel: The Fates of Human Societies*. New York: W.W. Norton.

Earle, L., Fozilhujaev, B., Tashbaeva, C. and Djamankulova, K. (2004) 'Community development in Kazakhstan, Kyrgyzstan and Uzbekistan', Occasional paper number 40. Oxford: INTRAC.

Eng, E. and Parker, E. (1994) 'Measuring community competence in the Mississippi delta: the interface between programme evaluation and empowerment', *Health Education Quarterly*, 21(2): 199–220.

Erzinger, S. (1994) 'Empowerment in Spanish: words can get in the way', *Health Education Quarterly*, 21(3): 417–19.

Everson, S. A., Lynch, J. W., Chesney, M. A., Kaplan, G. A., Goldberg, D. E., Shade, S. B., Cohen, R. D., Salonen, R. and Salonen, J. T. (1997) 'Interaction of workplace demands and cardiovascular reactivity in progression of carotid atherosclerosis: population based study', *British Medical Journal*, 314: 553–8.

Ewles, L. and Simnett, I. (2003) (fifth edition) *Promoting Health. A Practical Guide.* London: Bailliere Tindall.

Eyerman, R. and Jamison, A. (1991) *Social Movements. A Cognitive Approach.* Cambridge: Polity Press.

Faulkner, M. (2001) 'Empowerment and disempowerment: models of staff/patient interaction', *Nursing Times Research*, 6(6): 936–48.

Foucault, M. (1979) *Discipline and Punishment: The Birth of the Prison.* Middlesex: Peregrine Books.

Freeman, J. (ed.) (1983) *Social Movements of the Sixties and Seventies.* New York: Longman.

Freire, P. (1973) *Education for Critical Consciousness.* New York: Seabury Press.

Freudenberg, N. (1997) *Health Promotion in the City.* Atlanta. Centres for Disease Control and Prevention.

Gangolli, L. V., Duggal, R. and Shukla, A. (eds) (2005) *Review of Health Care in India.* Mumbai: CEHAT.

Gee, D. (2008) Park Scheme seeks more 'friends'. The Christchurch Press. www.bush.org.nz/library/934.html. accessed 3/4/2008.

Gibbon, M. (1999) Meetings with meaning: health dynamics in rural Nepal, unpublished PhD thesis. London: South Bank University.

Gibbon, M., Labonte, R. and Laverack, G. (2002) 'Evaluating community capacity', *Health and Social Care in the Community*, 10(6): 485–91.

Ginsberg, P. E. (1988) 'Evaluation in cross-cultural perspective', *Evaluation and Program Planning*, 11: 189–95.

Glesne, C. and Peshkin, A. (1992) *Becoming Qualitative Researchers.* New York: Longman Publishing Group.

Goodman, R. M., Speers, M. A., McLeroy, K., Fawcett, S., Kegler, M., Parker, E., Rathgeb Smith, S., Sterling, T. D. and Wallerstein, N. (1998) 'Identifying and Defining the Dimensions of Community Capacity to Provide a Basis for Measurement', *Health Education & Behavior*, 25(3): 258–78.

Gordon, G. (1995) 'Participation, empowerment and sexual health in Africa', in Craig, G. and Mayo, M. (eds) *Community Empowerment. A Reader in Participation and Development*, pp. 181–93. London: Zed Books.

Grace, V. M. (1991) 'The marketing of empowerment and the construction of the health consumer: a critique of health promotion', *International Journal of Health Services*, 21(2): 329–43.

Green, L. and Kreuter, M. (1991) *Health Promotion Planning. An Educational and Environmental Approach.* Toronto: Mayfield Publishing Company.

Hawe, P., King, L., Noort, M., Jordens, C. and Lloyd, B. (2000) Indicators to help with capacity building in health promotion. Sydney: Australian Centre for Health Promotion/NSW Health.

Haynes, A. W. and Singh, R. N. (1993) 'Helping families in developing countries: a model based on family empowerment and social justice', *Social Development Issues*, 15(1): 27–37.

Hubley, J. (1993) *Communicating Health: An Action Guide to Health Education and Health Promotion.* London: Macmillan.

Hunt, K., and Emslie, C. (2001) 'Commentary: the prevention paradox in lay epidemiology – Rose revisited', *International Journal of Epidemiology*, 30(3): 442–6.

IRED (1997) *People's Empowerment. Grassroots Experiences in Africa, Asia and Latin America.* Rome: IRED-NORD.

Israel, B. A., Checkoway, B., Schultz, A. and Zimmerman, M. (1994) 'Health education and community empowerment: conceptualizing and measuring perceptions of individual, organisational and community control', *Health Education Quarterly*, 21(2): 149–70.

Jackson, T., Mitchell, S. and Wright, M. (1989) 'The community development continuum', *Community Health Studies*, 8(1): 66–73.

Jones, A. and Laverack, G. (2003) 'Building Capable Communities within a Sustainable Livelihoods Approach: Experiences from Central Asia', http://www.livelihoods.org/lessons/Central Asia & Eastern Europe/SLLPC. 1.9.2003.

Jones, L. and Sidell, M. (eds) (1997) *The Challenge of Promoting Health. Exploration and Action.* London: Macmillan.

Jones, L., Sidell, M. and Douglas, J. (eds) (2002) *The Challenge of Promoting Health: Exploration and Action.* 2nd edition. London: Macmillan.

Kana'iaupuni, S. M. (2005) 'Ka'akalai Ku Kanaka: A call for strength-based approaches from a native Hawaiian perspective', *Educational Researcher*, 34(5): 32–8.

Kendall, S. (1998) (ed.) *Health and Empowerment: Research and Practice.* London: Arnold.

Kickbusch, I. (2002) The future of health promotion. http://info.med.yale.edu/eph/pdf/The%20Future%20of%20Health%20Promotion.pdf. Accessed 16/8/2007.

Kieffer, C. H. (1984) 'Citizen empowerment: a development perspective', *Prevention in Human Services*, 3: 9–36.

Kitzinger, J. (1995) 'Introducing focus groups', *British Medical Journal*, 311: 299–302.

Korsching, P. F. and Borich, T. O. (1997) 'Facilitating cluster communities: lessons from the Iowa experience', *Community Development Journal*, 32(4): 342–53.

Klawiter, M. (2004) 'Breast cancer in two regimes: the impact of social movements on illness experience', *Sociology of Health & Illness*, 26(6): 845–74.

Labonte, R. (1990) 'Empowerment: notes on professional and community dimensions', *Canadian Review of Social Policy*, 26: 64–75.

Labonte, R. (1993) Health Promotion and Empowerment: Practice Frameworks. Particip-ACTION. 3. Toronto: University of Toronto.

Labonte, R. (1994) 'Health promotion and empowerment: reflections on professional practice', *Health Education Quarterly*, 21(2): 253–68.

Labonte, R. (1996) Community development in the public health sector: the possibilities of an empowering relationship between the state and civil society, PhD thesis. Toronto: York University.

Labonte, R. (1998) A Community Development Approach to Health Promotion: A Background Paper on Practice Tensions, Strategic Models and Accountability Requirements for Health Authority Work on the Broad Determinants of Health. Edinburgh. Health Education Board for Scotland.

Labonte, R. and Laverack, G. (2008) *Health Promotion in Action: From Local to Global Empowerment.* London. Palgrave Macmillan.

Laverack, G. (1998) 'The concept of empowerment in a traditional Fijian context', *Journal of Community Health and Clinical Medicine for the Pacific*, 5(1): 26–9.

Laverack, G. (1999) Addressing the contradiction between discourse and practice in health promotion, unpublished PhD thesis. Melbourne: Deakin University.

Laverack, G. and Dap, H. D. (2004) 'Transforming information, education and communication in Vietnam', *Health Education*, 103(6): 363–9.

Laverack, G. and Labonte, R. (2000) 'A planning framework for the accommodation of community empowerment goals within health promotion programming', *Health Policy and Planning*, 15(3): 255–62.

Laverack, G. (2001) 'An identification and interpretation of the organizational aspects of community empowerment', *Community Development Journal*, 36(2): 40–52.

Laverack, G. and Thangphet, S. (2007) 'Building community capacity for locally managed ecotourism in Northern Thailand', *Community Development Journal*. Advanced access 14/11/2007. http://cdj.oxfordjournals.org/papbyrecent.dtl.

Laverack, G. (2003) 'Building capable communities: experiences in a rural Fijian context', *Health Promotion International*, 18(2): 99–106.

Laverack, G. and Brown, K. M. (2003) 'Qualitative research in a cross-cultural context: Fijian experiences', *Qualitative Health Research*, 13(3): 1–10.

Laverack, G. (2004) *Health Promotion Practice: Power and Empowerment*. London: Sage Publications.

Laverack, G. (2005) *Public Health: Power, Empowerment & Professional Practice*. London. Palgrave Macmillan.

Laverack, G. (2006) 'Using a "domains" approach to build community empowerment', *Community Development Journal*, 41(1): 4–12.

Laverack, G. 'Ofanoa, M., Nosa, V., Fa'alili, J. and Taufa, S. (2007) *Social and Cultural Perceptions of Community Empowerment in Four Pacific Peoples in Auckland, New Zealand*. New Zealand: The University of Auckland.

Laverack, G. (2007) *Health Promotion Practice: Building Empowered Communities*. London: Open University Press.

Laverack, G. (2008) The Future of Health Promotion Programming. Workshop presentation 'Empowerment for health promotion: Global experiences, German perspectives', Munich 21/1/2008.

Laverack, G., Hill, K., Akenson, L. and Corrie, R. (2009) *Building Capacity towards Health Leadership in Remote Indigenous Communities in Cape York*. Australian Indigenous HealthInfoNet. Vol. 9(1): 1–11. http://healthbulletin.org.au/articles/building-capacity-towards-health-leadership-in-remote-indigenous-communities-in-cape-york/ accessed 5/2/2009.

Lerner, M. (1986) *Surplus Powerlessness*. Oakland, CA.: The Institute for Labour and Mental Health.

Liew, T. (2007) *Glen Innes Household Needs Assessment*. New Zealand: University of Auckland.

Lloyd, M. and Bor, R. (2004) (second edition) *Communication Skills for Medicine*. London: Churchill Livingstone.

Loss, J. and Wise, M. (2007) *Concepts, Benefits and Limits of Empowerment and Participation in Community Based Health Promotion Practice – Results of a Qualitative Study*. Unpublished.

Lupton, D. (1995) *The Imperative of Health: Public Health and the Regulated Body*. London: Sage Publications.

MacPherson, D. W. and Gushulak, B. D. (2004) *Global Migration Perspectives. Global Commission on International Migration*. Geneva, Report Number 7, October 2004.

Manandhar, D. S., Osrin, D., Prasad Shrestha, B., Mesko, N., Morrison, J., Tumbahanghe, K. M., Tamang, S., Thapa, S., Shrestha, D., Thapa, B., Shrestha, J. R., Wade, A., Standing, H., Manandhar, M. M., de L. Costello, A. and members of the MIRA Makwanpur trial team (2004) 'Effect of a participatory intervention with women's groups on birth outcomes in Nepal: cluster-randomised controlled trial', *Lancet*, 364: 970–9.

Marsden, D., Oakley, P. and Pratt, B. (1994) *Measuring the Process: Guidelines for Evaluating Social Development*. Oxford: INTRAC.

Marshall, G. (1998) *A Dictionary of Sociology*. London: Oxford University Press.

Melucci, A. (1985) 'The symbolic challenge of contemporary movements', *Social Research*, 52(4): 789–816.

Merryfield, M. M. (1985) 'The challenge of cross-cultural evaluation: some views from the field', in Patton, M. Q. (ed.) *Culture and Evaluation*. San Francisco, C.A.: Jossey-Bass: 3–17.

Minichiello, V., Aroni, R., Timewell, E. and Alexander, L. (1990) *Indepth Interviewing. Researching People*. Australia: Longman Cheshire.

Ministry of Health (MoH, NZ, 2003) 'Project to counter stigma and discrimination associated with mental illness', *National Plan 2003–2005*. Wellington, New Zealand.

Mitchell, C. and Banks, M. (1998) *Handbook of Conflict Resolution. The Analytical Problem-Solving Approach*. London: Pinter.

Morriss, P. (1987) *Power. A Philosophical Analysis*. New York: St. Martin's Press.

National Strategic Framework for Aboriginal and Torres Strait Islander Health (2003) National Aboriginal and Torres Strait Islander Health Council, Context, NATSIHC, Canberra.

Nutbeam, D. (2000) 'Health literacy as a public health goal: a challenge for contemporary health education and communication strategies into the 21st century', *Health Promotion International*, 15(3): 259–67.

O'Connor, M. and Parker, E. (1995) *Health Promotion: Principles and Practice in the Australian Context*. St Leonards, NSW: Allen & Unwin Pty Ltd.

Pakulski, J. (1991) *Social Movements. The Politics of Moral Protest*. Sydney: Longman Cheshire.

Papa, M. J., Singhal, A. and Papa, W. H. (2006). *Organizing for Social Change: A Dialectic Journey of Theory and Praxis*. London: Sage Publications.

Photovoice (2008) Social change through photography. www.photovoice.com accessed 5/3/2008.

Piven, F. F. and Cloward, R. (1977) *Poor Peoples' Movements. Why they Succeed, How they Fail*. New York: Pantheon Books.

Rappaport, J. (1984) *Studies in Empowerment: Steps toward Understanding and Action*. New York: Haworth Press.

Rappaport, J. (1985) 'The power of empowerment language', *Social Policy*, Fall: 15–21.

Rappaport, J. (1987) 'Terms of empowerment/exemplars of prevention. Toward a theory of community psychology', *American Journal of Community Psychology*, 15: 121–47.

Raven, B. H. and Litman-Adizes, T. (1986) 'Interpersonal influence and social power in health promotion', in Ward, W. B. (ed.) *Advances in Health Education and Promotion*, pp. 181–209. London: Elsevier Science Ltd.

Renkert, S. and Nutbeam, D. (2001) 'Opportunities to improve maternal health literacy through antenatal education: an explanatory study', *Health Promotion International*, 16(4): 381–8.

Renewal.net (2008) resolving differences-building communities and Aik saath: Conflict resolution peer group facilitators. Renewal.net case studies. http://www.renewal.net/Documents/RNET/. Accessed 29/4/2008.

Rifkin, S. B. and Pridmore, P. (2001) *Partners in Planning: Information, Participation and Empowerment*. London: Macmillan Education.

Rifkin, S. B., Muller, F. and Bichmann, W. (1988) 'Primary health care: on measuring participation', *Social Science Medicine*, 9: 931–40.

Rissel, C. (1994) 'Empowerment: the holy grail of health promotion?', *Health Promotion International*, 9(1): 39–47.

Rissel, C., Perry, C. and Finnegan, J. (1996) 'Toward the assessment of psychological empowerment in health promotion: initial tests of validity and reliability', *Journal of the Royal Society of Health*, 116(4): 211–18.

Roberts, H. (1998) 'Empowering communities: the case of childhood accidents', in Kendall, S. (1998) (ed.) *Health and Empowerment: Research and Practice*. Chapter 6. London: Arnold.

Robertson, A. and Minkler, M. (1994) 'New health promotion movement: a critical examination', *Health Education Quarterly*, 21(3): 295–312.

Robson, C. (1993) *Real World Research*. Oxford: Blackwell Publishers Ltd.

Rose, G. (1985) 'Sick individuals and sick populations', *International Journal of Epidemiology*, 14: 32–8.

Roughan, J. J. (1986) Village organization for development, PhD thesis. Honolulu: Department of Political Science, University of Hawaii.

Russon, C. (1995) 'The influence of culture on evaluation', *Evaluation Journal of Australasia*, 7(1): 44–9.

Saskatoon Regional Health Authority (SRHA) (2005) *Saskatoon 'In motion': Five Years in the Making*. Saskatchewan. Saskatoon Regional Health Authority.

Scrambler, G. (1987) 'Habermas and the power of medical expertise', in Scrambler, G. (ed.) *Sociological Theory and Medical Sociology*. New York: Methuen Press.

Scrimgeour, D. (1997) 'Community control of aboriginal health services in the Northern Territory'. Darwin: Menzies School of Health Research, 2/97.

Seefeldt, F. M. (1985) 'Cultural considerations for evaluation consulting in the Egyptian context', in Patton, M. Q. (ed.) *Culture and Evaluation.* San Francisco, CA.: Jossey-Bass: 69–78.

Seidman, S. and Wagner, D. G. (eds) (1992) *Postmodernism and Social Theory. The Debate Over General Theory.* Oxford: Blackwell.

Seligman, M. (1975) *Helplessness: On Depression, Development and Death.* San Francisco, CA.: W. H. Freeman.

Serrano-Garcia, I. (1984) 'The illusion of empowerment: community development within a colonial context', in Rappaport, J. (eds) *Studies in Empowerment: Steps toward Understanding Action.* New York: Haworth Press: 173–200.

Shrimpton, R. (1995) 'Community participation in food and nutrition programmes: an analysis of recent governmental experiences', in Pinstrup-Andersen, P., Pellitier, D. and Alderman, H. (eds) *Child Growth and Nutrition in Developing Countries: Priorities for Action.* USA, Ithaca: Cornell University Press: 243–61.

Simpson, G. E. and Yinger, J. M. (1965) *Racial and Cultural Minorities.* New York: Harper and Row.

Small, C. (1999) 'Finding an invisible history', *Journal of Artificial Societies and Social Simulation,* 2: 3.

Smith, R. (2002) 'The discomfort of patient power', *British Medical Journal,* 324: 497–8.

Speer, P. and Hughley, J. (1995) 'Community organising. an ecological route to empowerment and power', *American Journal of Community Psychology,* 23(5): 729–48.

Srinivasan, L. (1993) *Tools for Community Participation. A Manual for Training Trainers in Participatory Techniques.* New York: PROWWESS/UNDP.

Starhawk, M. S. (1990) *Truth or Dare. Encounters with Power, Authority and Mystery.* New York: HarperCollins.

Statistics New Zealand (2007) QuickStats about culture and identity. Wellington, New Zealand. www.stats.govt.nz/census/2006-census-data/quickstats-about-culture-identity/quickstats-about-culture-and-identity.htm, 2 September 2008 [date last accessed].

Stewart, M. A., Brown, J. B., Weston, W. W., et al. (2003) *Patient Centred Medicine: Transforming the Clinical Method. 2nd Edition.* Oxford. Radcliffe Medical Publications.

Stewart, D. W. and Shamdasani, P. N. (1990) *Focus Groups. Theory and Practice.* London: Sage Publications.

Swift, C. and Levin, G. (1987) 'Empowerment: an emerging mental health technology', *Journal of Primary Prevention,* 8(1 and 2): 71–94.

Syme, L. (1997) 'Individual vs community interventions in public health practice: some thoughts about a new approach', *Vichealth Letter,* July(2): 2–9.

Taylor, V. (1995) 'Social reconstruction and community development in the transition to democracy in South Africa', in Craig, G. and Mayo, M. (eds) *Community Empowerment: A Reader in Participation and Development,* pp. 168–80. London: Zed Books.

Tengland, P. (2007) 'Empowerment: a goal or a means for health promotion?', *Medicine, Health Care and Philosophy,* 10: 197–207.

Thangphet, S. (2006) Building capacity of community ecotourism for income generation and biodiversity conservation in Northern Thailand. Nagao Natural Environment Foundation. Chang Mai. Thailand.

Tse, S., Laverack, G., Nayar, S. and Foroughian, S. (2008) 'Community engagement for health promotion: Reducing injuries among Chinese people in New Zealand', *Health Education Journal,* forthcoming.

Turbyne, J. (1996) The Enigma of Empowerment: A Study of the Transformation of Concepts in Policy Making Processes, PhD. Bath: University of Bath.

Untamed Path (2007) 'What is Ecotourism?', http://www.untamedpath.com/Ecotourism/what_is_ecotourism.html. P. 1. Accessed 28/6/2007.

Uphoff, N. (1991) 'A field methodology for participatory self-education', *Community Development Journal,* 26(4): 271–85.

Victurine, R. (2000) 'Building tourism excellence at the community level: capacity building for community-based entrepreneurs in Uganda', *Journal of Travel Research*, 38(3): 221–9.

Wang, C. C. and Pies, C. A. (2004) 'Family, maternal and child health through photo-voice', *Maternal and Child Health Journal*, 8(2): 95–102.

Wanless, D. (2003) *Securing Good Health for the Whole Population: Population Health Trends*. London: HMSO.

Ward, J. (1987) 'Community development with marginal people: the role of conflict', *Community Development Journal*, 22(1): 18–21.

Wartenberg, T. E. (1990) *The Forms of Power. From Domination to Transformation*. Philadelphia, PA.: Temple University Press.

Werner, D. (1988) 'Empowerment and health', *Contact, Christian Medical Commission*, 102: 1–9.

Westwood, J. and Brous, D. (1993) 'Cross-cultural evaluation: lessons from experience', *Evaluation Journal of Australasia*, 5(1): 43–8.

Wharf-Higgins, J., Naylor, P. J. and Day, M. (2007) 'Seed funding for health promotion: sowing sustainability or scepticism?', *Community Development Journal*. Advance access January 31, 2007, pp. 1–12.

Wheat, S. (1997) 'Banking on a better future', *Guardian Weekly*, Manchester, February 9: 19.

Wood, S., Sawyer, R. and Simpson-Hebert, M. (1998) *PHAST Step-by-step-Guide*. Geneva: WHO.

World Health Organisation (1978) *Declaration of Alma Ata*. Geneva: WHO.

World Health Organisation (1986) *Ottawa Charter for Health Promotion*. Geneva: WHO.

World Health Organisation (1998) *Health Promotion Glossary*. Geneva. WHO.

World Health Organisation (2005) The Bangkok Charter for Health Promotion in a Globalized World. 6th Global Conference on Health Promotion. Bangkok, Thailand. World Health Organisation. http://www.who.int/healthpromotion/conferences/6gchp/bangkok_charter/en. 22/5/2006.

WHO (2007) Operationalising empowerment to improve maternal and newborn health: a guide to the workshop for Maternal and Newborn Health programme managers and providers. Geneva: World Health Organisation (unpublished report).

Wrong, D. H. (1988) *Power. Its Forms, Bases and Uses*. Chicago, IL.: The University of Chicago Press.

Zakus, J. D. L. and Lysack, C. L. (1998) 'Revisiting community participation', *Health Policy and Planning*, 13(1): 1–12.

Zimmerman, M. A. and Rappaport, J. (1988) 'Citizen participation, perceived control and psychological empowerment', *American Journal of Community Psychology*, 16(5): 725–43.

Zimmerman, M. A. and Zahniser, J. H. (1991) 'Refinements of sphere-specific measures of perceived control: development of a socio-political control scale', *Journal of Community Psychology*, 19: 189–204.

Index